YOUR
HEALING
POWER

Also by Jack Angelo

Spiritual Healing: Energy Medicine for Today

YOUR HEALING POWER

A Comprehensive Guide to Channelling Your Healing Energies

JACK ANGELO

PIATKUS

ACKNOWLEDGEMENTS

I would like to thank my wife, Jan, for her support, inspiration and painstaking work at all stages of the book; Estella White who, over the years, has given much to healing and to us; Shirley Brooker; all my patients and workshop participants who have taught me so much about the human spirit.

Names and situations have been changed in the case histories to protect privacy.

First published in 1994 by
Judy Piatkus (Publishers) Ltd of
5 Windmill Street, London W1P 1HF

Reprinted 1995

The moral right of the author has been asserted

*A catalogue record for this book is available
from the British Library*

ISBN 0-7499-1326-6 pb

Illustrations by Taurus Graphics

Set in Linotron Century O.S. by
Computerset Ltd, Harmondsworth
Printed and bound in Great Britain by
Butler & Tanner Ltd, Frome

Contents

The Exercises

There is a sacred journey we were born to undertake.
It is the Great Healing.

Stephen Levine in *Guided Meditations,*
Explorations and Healings

Introduction

*I*t was my first night in San Gimignano. All was quiet in the Fanciulli's house where I had rented a room. I lay awake planning the research I was to do in the coming month. Suddenly a rasping sound broke the silence. The old grandfather was coughing. On and on he coughed until the cough changed to groans and cries of desperation. The rest of the house was still. No one went to his aid. Perhaps the family slept through it because they were used to these harrowing sounds and felt powerless to bring him any form of relief.

I wanted to help him. I was lying on my back and something made me put my hands outside the bedclothes. Straight away I felt the palms and fingertips tingling. I mentally asked for help to be sent to the old man. The next moment his coughing stopped as if cut off. The house was quiet again.

In the small hours of the next night the old man began to cough, hardly able to pause for breath, until it seemed he would cough up his whole body. Again I stretched out my hands and asked for help for him. The coughing stopped immediately and he was able to get a good night's sleep.

The same thing happened every night until I left San Gimignano. It was my first attempt at distant healing and I had discovered that whatever made my hands tingle could be sent somewhere to help someone.

On my return to Britain, I joined a local meditation group. The leader sensed that I had the 'gift of healing' and I was asked to send distant healing to various people. I was not told how to do this so I had to work it out my own way, intuitively.

When I sat quietly to do this, I could 'feel' each person in front of me and sometimes 'see' the body from whatever angle was necessary. I knew where on the body I was placing my hands and what was wrong with the organs concerned. I often 'saw' or 'felt' what was taking place as the healing progressed. In this way I was able to work with people as if they were physically present.

During the ensuing weeks, feedback from many of those who had requested my help gave me proof that distant healing was effective for all kinds of conditions.

This is how I started healing so that I felt quite confident by the time I came to work 'hands-on'. I would know where to put my hands and found that I could pick up a range of messages coming from different parts of a person's body. These told me not only of the physical conditions, but of worries, sadness, pressures, past traumas, life incidents, unfulfilled needs, as if everything that had happened to that person, everything that they were thinking and feeling was recorded somewhere in their body. Just like a radio set, if I 'tuned in' I could receive the relevant information.

MY FIRST ENCOUNTER WITH A HEALER

In my case these abilities, which all of us possess to varying degrees, were 'switched on' by the experiences of chronic illness. Some months before my trip to Italy I went to see a spiritual healer as a last resort on the recommendation of a friendly editor.

Amazingly, my disabling sciatica and back trouble was almost completely healed after two sessions. With hindsight I know that I was in a state of readiness and that part of me expected the healing to take place.

I was also sceptical as well as curious. Healing worked. But how? Where did it come from? What part had the healer played? My questions were met with the disarming reply: 'It's the power of love. It comes from God, through me and into you. This gets your own healing power working. But you can't heal someone you don't like.' In the charged atmosphere of the healing session, the idea of *love* as an energy which could heal was exciting and not at all naive. I knew this simple yet powerful concept was right.

It was my first encounter with a healer and I had been fortunate. Carl Jung would have called our meeting 'synchronistic' in that it played a big part in changing my life. Before I left I asked the healer his opinion about my becoming a healer too. He laughed and said, 'I think it would be a great idea!' I was given no instructions, just the assurance that I would be guided. His parting words were: 'You'll never be the same again now spirit has touched you.'

This phenomenon of spirit touching me and touching others, what this touch is, its effects and why we need it, has been the focus of my life ever since.

I feel that I was born knowing how to heal, that the ability was always close to the surface. As a child, no one needed to tell me what to do because healing had no name. It was something I just did as naturally as running, jumping, singing and playing. I enjoyed the company of old people, those who were sick or even dying.

In my teens and twenties, healing more often took the form of simply being a sympathetic listener, or of taking time out with society's losers and underdogs. Occasionally people asked for hands-on help, but I never thought of it as an ability I could develop or use to benefit others.

When the reawakening came, it was as if I could plug into a knowledge bank which had just been reactivated after a period of dormancy. But, apart from the writings of Harry Edwards, there were few books around which could confirm my own findings. However, I was fortunate in making two friends who were wonderful healers and who were well-developed spiritually as well as physically. I used them as sounding boards, listening and learning. I was also aware that learning was taking place in other ways and with other teachers. For example, I would awake to recall sessions of instruction which had occurred in the dream state.

Nevertheless, at that time I would have welcomed a book on the subject which brought together the many strands of knowledge under one cover. I would have liked to explore information about the human body and its subtle aspects, the aura and the energy centres, how the energies of healing work, and I would have wanted all this liberally laced with how-to-do-it exercises to broaden my practical experience. The gift of healing cannot be taught but it can certainly be awakened and developed through careful training.

A COMPREHENSIVE PRACTICAL GUIDE

Your Healing Power has been created in response to the need I experienced when I started healing. Through my meetings with other healers and people on workshops and training courses I recognize that this need is not peculiar to me. This book is a comprehensive and practical guide for those who wish to explore the subject, for those who wish to work on themselves and for those who wish to work as healers.

The physical body is seen as part of an interrelated system of other subtle bodies which is your whole being. The exercises help you to develop an understanding of the system and to work efficiently with its energies.

The healer also needs to understand the nature of disease, the role of the mind and emotions, how healing relates to birth and death as well as to ill health. Further exercises will give you hands-on experience of all these aspects and insight into how you function as a multi-dimensional being.

Finally, detailed instructions on the act of healing, ways of working and how to run a healing practice will equip you to take the work a stage further. The book can therefore be used as a self-healing manual, a guidance manual for healers and as a workshop text.

THE HISTORICAL PERSPECTIVE

If you wonder when and where spiritual healing began, just think about the fact that it is the most natural thing to put a hand over the place which is hurting. It may be over your own body, someone else's, an animal's body, a plant or a part of the living earth. This universal impulse arises from the truth that the hand has the power to heal. It is the basis of all healing.

Throughout history the healer was singled out as one who seemed particularly gifted at directing healing energies. This probably led to the creation of healing and later medicine as a trade, which was an art as well as a craft, later a science and a profession. But the progress towards the profession of physician meant that the role of healer began to change from one who helped you get in touch with your own healing power to one who helped you give it up to an expert. Two important historical developments allowed this to happen.

In ancient times there was no division between body, mind and spirit so that energy was understood as a force which permeated this trinity. All things originated from the same spiritual source and this was the same source of healing energies. But with the development of science and the shift in religious outlook, particularly in the west, certain things came to be designated spiritual, or of the spirit world, while the rest were clearly material, of the physical world. The two worlds, instead of penetrating each other and mingling with each other, became separated.

The second development, within Christendom, was the outlawing of healing outside of the Church and the systematic execution of lay healers and psychics. The impact of centuries of such persecution has been so powerful that even today there is much ignorance and fear surrounding our healing birthright. This attitude of prejudice also led to the disastrous policy of repression of ancient healing techniques wherever Christianity has been imposed throughout the world.

The legacy of these historical events has meant that medicine and health care have evolved without a spiritual base, with attitudes to human beings and illness derived from current scientific thinking alone. By the seventeenth century, the Newtonian world view encouraged doctors to think of us as a series of mechanical systems controlled by a bio-computer, the brain. The soul part of us – if it existed at all – was the domain of the Church. The coming of the Industrial Revolution in the eighteenth century, driven by scientific inventions, caused many thinkers to question the direction in which materialism was leading. Machines could be destructive and enslaving as well as beneficial. In the advancement of humankind something was missing and, despite the presence of the Church in every village it seemed to be the spiritual dimension. The artist and poet William Blake (1757 – 1827), for example, saw the new mills as 'dark' and 'satanic' and he asserted that 'man has no body distinct from his soul, for that called body is a portion of soul discerned by the senses . . .' William Wordsworth and his sister Dorothy both sought in their writings to emphasize the spiritual basis of life and nature which they felt was being overlooked in favour of material progress.

It was a time during which people were looking for freedom of all kinds, particularly of the spirit. Not surprisingly perhaps, psychic and spiritual awareness had reached a peak. This manifested in the United States with the opening up of communication between psychically aware people and those existing on subtler levels of being (so-called 'spirit people'). These subtle beings assured those who were able to tune in to them that within the coming 150 years the phenomenon of psychic awareness would become worldwide and occur amongst all peoples. The gift of healing would be returned to the people and would soon be powerfully demonstrated. This would be accompanied by a reawakening of true spirituality which would herald a new age.

It was not long before these predictions were confirmed, but healing was still outlawed beyond the Church setting (only becoming legal in 1951). The founding of the spiritualist religion provided a place where healing could be practised legally, along with clairvoyance and other mediumistic abilities. Healing owes a debt to spiritualism for fostering its development, but, in the public mind, this has led to the association of spiritual healing with the beliefs and practices of spiritualism. The fact is that some healers are spiritualists but many are not.

With the pioneering work of great healers such as Harry Edwards, who brought healing into the public domain during the first half of this century, healing developed rapidly. Before his death, Edwards founded the National Federation of Spiritual Healers (NFSH) which is now the largest healing organization in the world, and is strictly non-denominational (see under Useful Addresses). It has affiliated associations in America, Canada, Australia, New Zealand, South Africa and Ireland.

The Confederation of Healing Organizations (CHO), and more recently the British Complementary Medicine Association (BCMA), are the umbrella bodies to which most healing organizations in the UK belong. They have come to be the negotiating voice with orthodox medicine, government and with the European Community, where healing is still illegal in some countries. These bans are largely due to long-standing religious and medical ignorance about the nature of healing energies.

The historical legacy of the divorce between spirit and life is, of course, not just an issue which healers have to face. We have all been conditioned by a culture which has accepted and promoted this divorce as a fact of life. But the process of linking all therapies and medicine to the concept of oneness, the concept of holism, has begun.

In the UK many doctors employ healers as part of the range of services being offered to patients. Health care professionals now attend healing workshops and training courses and training programmes in spiritual healing have been specially developed by the NFSH for this group.

Research programmes in the USA, such as those carried out by the University of Colorado, are encouraging American physicians to look more closely at the potential for spiritual healing in medical practice. In Russia, the successful pioneering work of Clif and Galina Sanderson, with victims of radioactive fallout, has the full support of the scientific and medical establishment.

A POWERFUL COMPLEMENTARY THERAPY

Throughout the world there have been tremendous changes in people's lives during the last five years and this is reflected in the changes through which spiritual healing has been going. My own practice shows that personal and relationship problems, mental, emotional and spiritual dilemmas, as well as physical illness, are all conditions to which healing can effectively be applied. It is no longer a last resort but recognizably a powerful complementary therapy.

Just as illness brought me to healing, it made me aware of the need for total wholeness. I wonder what has brought you to this book? Is it a personal trauma, a crisis, general interest, a response to the apparent disintegration of society or are you driven by the desire to help? Even if you are just sceptical but curious, you will find something here to interest you, to set you thinking, perhaps even practising. But remember – you will never be the same again once healing has touched you!

How to Use
This Book

This book has evolved out of my years of practice as a healer and workshop facilitator and includes all the material given on my training courses.

The exercises are carefully structured so that they provide an enjoyable way of absorbing and understanding the information through practical experience. You may find it easier to tape the instructions for the exercises so that you do not have to refer to the text. This will avoid you breaking concentration and interrupting the process of the exercise.

Each chapter of the book builds on what has already been practised so spend as much time as you need before moving on to the next topic. Some exercises may seem easier to carry out than others. Remember that all your practice is helping to awaken and develop your awareness so that the process of each exercise is as important as the end result.

Keep practising what you are good at, what you enjoy and what comes naturally and don't be disheartened if some 'results' seem elusive at first. You can always go back to repeat an exercise with the benefit of the experience you have acquired. This is also an excellent way to monitor your progress.

A faculty of the mind which many of the book's exercises use is the imagination, or more accurately the ability to *visualize* something. We all have this ability and we use it every time we create something new. Even things like planning your day, choosing what to wear, organizing a meal or party, involve your ability to visualize. But when people come to use this natural faculty of the mind to help themselves, some find it very difficult. My advice is – do not ever worry if you cannot 'see' as directed in the context of an exercise. The exercise is carried out through the power of your mind. The mental command will mean that it has taken place. Once you relax and allow your natural faculties to operate, blocks to experience will dissolve.

As you work through the book, it's a good idea to keep a journal. Make notes on what you do and when, as well as the outcome. Put in relevant comments, insights and dreams, and anything else you wish, to enrich the log of your progress.

If you cannot find the words to express your experiences, try illustrating them or expressing them in some other way.

If you use the book for group work, keep a note of what happens to participants and how they respond to the material.

AN ADVENTURE IN AWARENESS

As you work through the exercises in the order given, you will notice a change in your perceptions. This may take the form of heightened sensitivity or a broader range of what you perceive, or both. You may also feel more confident and balanced within yourself. An attitude of open-mindedness and positive expectation will enhance your enjoyment of the material. Experiment and keep notes of your results. Self-discovery can be fun and learning to be aware of and trust your perceptions is an adventure.

As healers develop their abilities and ways of working, they find that personal transformation is as much a part of the process. You can therefore expect issues of personal development to surface as you progress through the material. For this reason I recommend that you work with a trustworthy partner or a group under the guidance of an experienced facilitator. If you decide to work alone, find a healer or a healing group nearby to whom you can refer and discuss your experiences (see Useful Addresses).

Your Healing Power can be used as a course of training in self-healing as well as healing development for healers and other therapists.

On completion of the course, as recommended, you will have equipped yourself with a powerful self-healing strategy. You will be much more aware of your own systems. You will be able to identify imbalance and you will be able to correct this imbalance or disharmony. Once you have learned how to help yourself you will be in a better position to help others. This book will provide you with the framework you need to function as a healer, safely, effectively, and with confidence.

1

The Physical Body

I *had called to see an elderly woman in some newly-built sheltered housing. Her husband explained that his wife had been suffering from chronic arthritis for many years, and the most painful area was the left hip. She lay down as comfortably as she could and I put my hands over the hip. It immediately began taking in energy. At first, the old lady seemed relaxed, then she suddenly became distressed. I held her hand.*

'What are you thinking about?' I asked her. 'Is something coming into your mind?'

With that she broke into deep sobs and wept for a few minutes. As her tears fell, I felt a dramatic increase in the level of energy being absorbed by her hip. After some 10 minutes, the flow decreased and she lay back against the pillows, breathing deeply.

When she was a girl of 14 she had been sent from her home in South Wales to work as a servant at a large house in Surrey. During the healing she saw the scene again quite vividly. Both she and her mother were crying bitterly over the separation to come. For two years she could not go home and she was very unhappy to be so far away from her family.

It seemed that she had stored much of her anger and sorrow in her hip, for the pain was almost completely cleared after the first healing session. I had been called to deal with a problem in someone's physical body only to find that healing released feelings that were generated nearly 70 years

> *before. This release played an important part in clearing up the crippling arthritis from which she had been suffering.*
>
> *In its great wisdom, her body had stored the repressed energies in certain weak areas in her skeleton. In her case, the stored energies attracted the deposition of chemicals which built up over the years so that the day came when she was forced to address the pain. Medication had helped up to a point, but the pain ensured that she would not be able to mask the underlying cause of it.*

The lesson for me is that the body is more than a set of physical systems, and obviously closely linked with other energies connected to thought and feeling. Furthermore, as well as carrying out its normal functions, it finds ways to signal to us when balance is disturbed on other levels of life – the emotional, mental and spiritual. And it does this in a physical way through its own structure.

GETTING TO KNOW YOUR BODY

You need to know about your body because through it you, as a soul, experience, learn and live your life. Since you are so intimately related to it you should get to know it as well as you can.

For healers, knowledge of the body and the language of health care allows us to draw closer to the medical profession who, until comparatively recently, have shouldered the total responsibility for the nation's health and wellbeing. In doing so, we can learn to speak the same language for we are all here for the same reason, the benefit of the patient.

Last, but not least, knowledge of the body is needed because it is what the patient usually presents to the healer. And this arises out of the body's ability to draw our attention to disharmony of any kind.

PATTERNS OF ENERGY

If you could break down your body into small units, you would find it composed of millions of cells. If these were further broken down into molecules, then atoms, you would end up with the smallest of units, the subatomic particles, all of which are vibrating patterns of energy.

The first exercise encourages you to think of yourself and other people as beings of energy, as patterns of living light. As you will find later, the pattern of light, which is you, is a combination of many vibrations. These vibrations emanate an energy which can be sensed by another person. We are all sensing each other in this way, though we may not be conscious of it. By working with the exercises in this book, you will develop your awareness so that it becomes conscious.

EXERCISE 1: Looking for the Light Around People

○ When you are with other people, see if you notice the aura of light projecting an inch or so from their body. It shows up particularly around the head (the halo). This is an emanation from within. The whole person is vibrating with energy. As you are observing a number of people at the same time, make a note of any perceived differences. Are there any links between the quality and/or quantity of light around a person and their mood or appearance? Don't worry if you do not see anything at your first few attempts, the key to seeing in this way is to relax.

THE NETWORK OF CONSCIOUSNESS

Ancient wisdom always taught that human bodies were patterns of energy, that matter and energy are one and the same. Furthermore, because all energy originates from the Source of consciousness, energy is conscious. This has important implications for healing, for it follows that each energy pattern will be conscious, whether it is a particle, a cell, an organ or a complete physical body. It also follows that every unit of energy within a large pattern, such as an organ, will be in touch with each other through what I call *the network of consciousness*.

Since Einstein formulated his general theory of relativity in 1916, physicists have discovered that subatomic particles behave in singular ways. For example, their movement is influenced by the one who is observing them. The consciousness of subatomic particles is affected by the energies being directed to them in the form of thought.

The striking fact that thought influences matter at an energetic level supports the findings of holistic healing that mind and the emotions have a profound effect on the harmony of the body. For they can alter the behaviour of its minutest components, the very energies which go to build its structure and compose its interrelated systems.

THE FUNDAMENTAL UNIT OF LIFE

The cell is the fundamental unit in all physical forms of human, animal and plant (Fig. 1). Its complex operations (considered by biologists to be the living process) are linked through the network of consciousness and driven by the life force. Everything that happens in the body occurs as a result of the organized and co-ordinated activities of the cells. When these activities are not co-ordinated for the benefit of the whole, diseases such as cancer are produced.

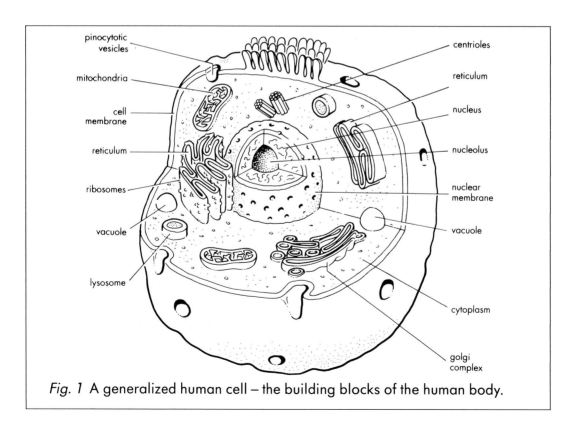

Fig. 1 A generalized human cell – the building blocks of the human body.

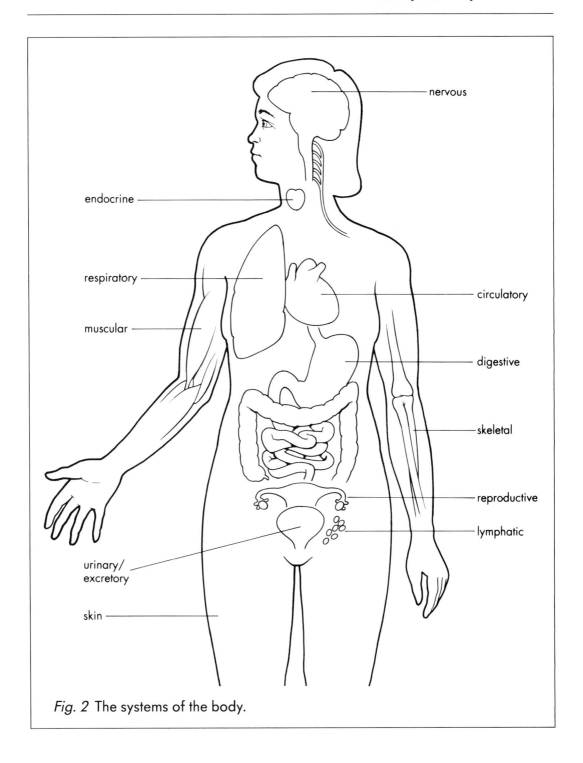

Fig. 2 The systems of the body.

THE SYSTEMS OF THE PHYSICAL BODY

When the cells act together to form organs and tissues they form the various systems which make up the 'temple of the soul'.

Each of the systems shown in Fig. 2 acts in a co-ordinated way to ensure the smooth functioning of your body. By getting to know your body, you will come to understand the fine balance of its systems, to honour it and to become more *positively* involved with it. Perhaps you hardly think about it until illness or disturbance strikes. Then suddenly it is the centre of your attention, like the friend whom you only contact when you want something from them.

At such times, because you focus on the part which is causing you to notice it, you think of parts of your body or its systems in isolation. But they should always be seen as elements of an integrated whole. Furthermore, your body is in a state of balance or imbalance with all your subtle bodies, which will be discussed later.

Healing will make you much more conscious of your hands and the energies which they can sense and transmit. Many of the exercises will increase your 'hand consciousness' and the sensitivity of your hands. In the following exercise, let's see just how sensitive your hands are as you begin to work with this first part of the book.

EXERCISE 2: Sensing Your Hands' Energies

○ Stand or sit comfortably. Take three breaths to energize yourself.

○ Hold your hands up to about waist height, with the palms facing inwards, and the width of your body between them. Let the hands relax so that the fingers separate naturally. Notice what you sense.

○ Being them together slowly, again noticing what you sense as you do so (Fig. 3).

○ Now rub your hands together briskly and hold them out again as before. Bring them together slowly, noticing what you sense as you do so.

○ Rub your hands together and hold them out again, this time with twice the width between them. Bring them together slowly. What do you notice?

○ Finally, rub your hands together and hold them out as far as you can. Bring them together slowly. Did you find a difference in what you sensed?

You may have sensed the energies of your hands as something like a soft ball between them, which grew in size as you rubbed your hands together each time. If you are wondering why this should be so, the first clue comes in Chapter 4.

○ Now work the same way again, but with a partner to see what you can sense together.

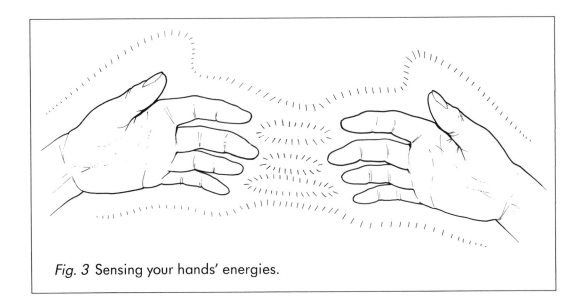

Fig. 3 Sensing your hands' energies.

EXERCISE 3: Sensing the Hands' Energies with a Partner

○ Stand opposite your partner with an arm's length between you.

○ Both rub your hands together briskly and hold them at shoulder height with the palms facing your partner.

○ Close your eyes.

○ Slowly move your two palms towards each other. Notice what you sense.

○ Stop when you can feel your palms 'bouncing' gently against the 'ball' of energy between you. Open your eyes and see where your hands are.

○ Now stand six paces apart and rub your hands together.

○ Close your eyes. Hold your hands up in the same way as before and slowly step towards your partner until you can sense the ball of energy again.

○ Open your eyes and see if the ball of energy you are both sensing has grown bigger.

○ Finally, stand twelve paces apart and repeat the sensing with your eyes closed. Discuss with your partner what you both sensed.

○ Decide whether you think you could go on increasing the distance between you and what the reason for this might be.

These exercises have given you a taste of things to come, as far as your hands are concerned. Now we will return to linking with the body consciousness.

One of the important functions of the body is to provide the soul with a vehicle for travelling on the Earth plane. The bony skeleton is the framework of the vehicle and the muscles allow the skeleton to move (Fig. 4). The form of the body is given largely by the muscles.

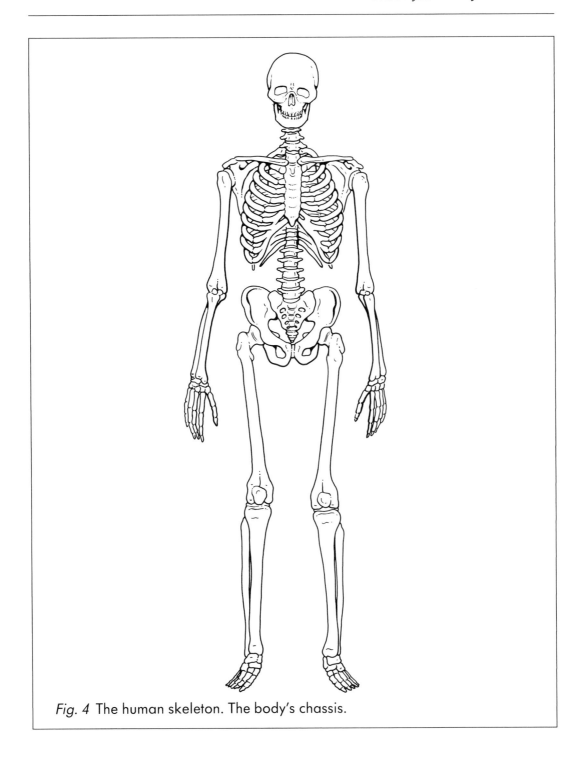

Fig. 4 The human skeleton. The body's chassis.

The Circulatory System

The muscles need large amounts of oxygen and nutrients to function efficiently. Such life-sustaining materials are carried to all the tissues via the flow of blood throughout the body. The flow is kept going by the heart which acts like a pump. Arteries carry oxygenated blood to the cells and carry all blood away from the heart. The veins carry all blood *to* the heart. The circulatory system is one of the most important networks of the body (Fig. 5).

The blood also conveys the subtle energy of the life force to all the cells. Blood has always been treated with respect since ancient times and we know that it is the liquid of life. The ritual of becoming blood brother or sister can elevate a person above even the ties of family relationship.

Blood has a deep and powerful meaning for us. In some societies the menstrual flow in women signals a time of significant surge in female power. By relaxing and communicating with blood and the heart we may discover much which will add to our understanding of life and each other.

If all energy patterns are conscious, it should be possible for us to link up with our own network of consciousness. The next exercise asks you to see the blood as a tissue which has no limiting form, like your heart, but which has a consciousness with which you can link. Blood has the form of flow and motion and it is one of the great energy patterns which streams through your body.

EXERCISE 4: Following the Blood

○ Sit or lie quietly and relax. Breathe slowly and gently.

○ Think of your blood system. Oxygenated blood has a vital, red colour. In your mind's eye, see it flowing round your body, transporting all the various materials to and from the cells, quietly and efficiently. Now focus on a part of your body. Visualize the red blood flowing in like liquid light to nourish and sustain this part.

If you are injured or in pain, see the blood bringing help and comfort to the affected parts. It is good also, whenever you practise this exercise, to send a thought of gratitude for the work the blood is doing on your behalf. Remember, it is bringing the life force itself to every cell.

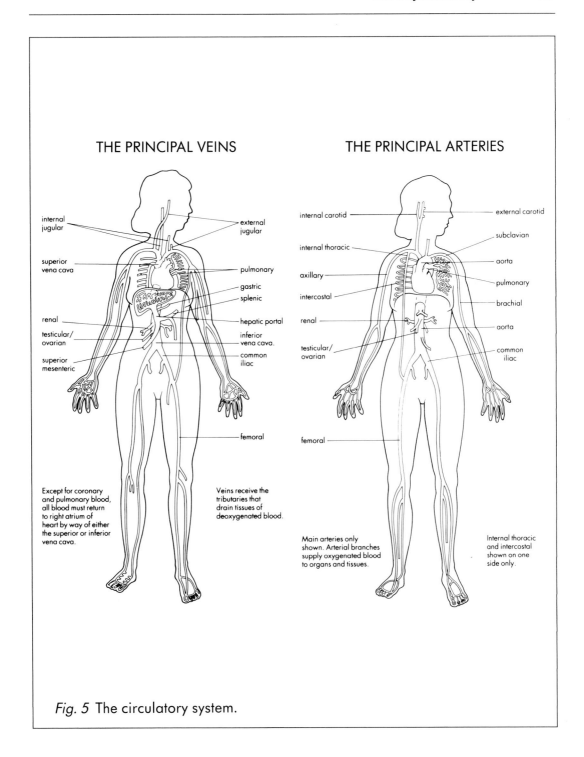

THE PRINCIPAL VEINS

internal jugular
external jugular
superior vena cava
pulmonary
gastric
splenic
renal
hepatic portal
testicular/ovarian
inferior vena cava.
superior mesenteric
common iliac
femoral

Except for coronary and pulmonary blood, all blood must return to right atrium of heart by way of either the superior or inferior vena cava.

Veins receive the tributaries that drain tissues of deoxygenated blood.

THE PRINCIPAL ARTERIES

internal carotid
external carotid
internal thoracic
subclavian
aorta
axillary
pulmonary
intercostal
brachial
renal
aorta
testicular/ovarian
common iliac
femoral

Main arteries only shown. Arterial branches supply oxygenated blood to organs and tissues.

Internal thoracic and intercostal shown on one side only.

Fig. 5 The circulatory system.

EXERCISE 5: Following the Heart

○ Sit or lie down quietly and relax. Breathe slowly and rhythmically.

○ Allow the mind to gently rest on the heart. Visualize your heart carrying out its work in an aura of tranquility. As you breathe calmly in and out, so your heart beats with the same calm rhythm. It, too, needs the nourishment of your positive and loving thoughts.

EXERCISE 6: For Women

Menstruation is a time of heightened sensitivity. This is a unique and rhythmic occurrence during which you can acknowledge and get in touch with the power that is specially yours.

○ Give yourself time and space to be quiet and passive.

○ Then, if you wish, enter into a dialogue with different parts of your body during this special time.

○ Keep a record of this communication in your journal. It will be very interesting to watch its development as you work with the course material.

The Lymphatic System

The body is largely composed of fluids. Those other than blood ultimately drain into the veins via the lymphatic system (Fig. 6). This consists of fluid compartments which assist the veins in draining many of the body tissues. Lymph nodes are part of the network of lymphatic tissue which, along with the spleen, thymus gland and tonsils, plays a leading role in the body's defence system. When any of the network becomes painful or enlarged, the system is

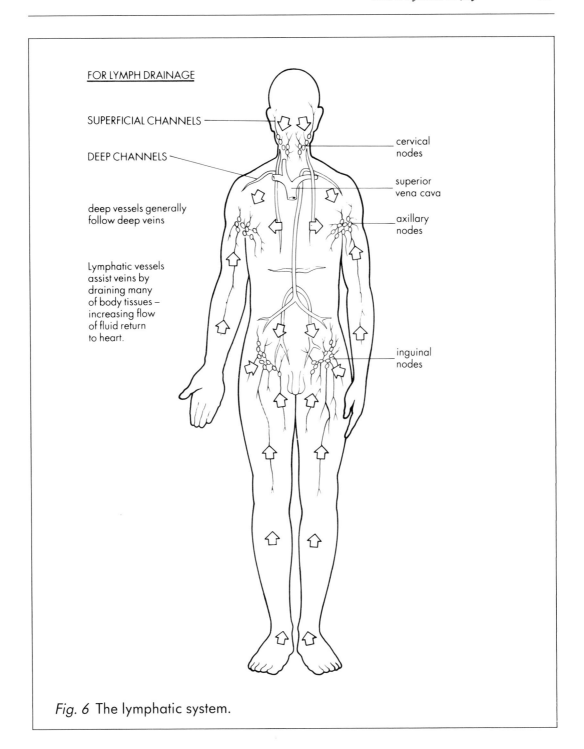

FOR LYMPH DRAINAGE

SUPERFICIAL CHANNELS

DEEP CHANNELS

deep vessels generally
follow deep veins

Lymphatic vessels
assist veins by
draining many
of body tissues –
increasing flow
of fluid return
to heart.

cervical
nodes

superior
vena cava

axillary
nodes

inguinal
nodes

Fig. 6 The lymphatic system.

probably having difficulty in dealing with destructive organisms such as bacteria.

The Digestive System

You need physical nourishment in the form of food and water. The digestive system allows you to process these and to extract what the body requires. The excretory system allows you to get rid of waste products from this process and from other bodily activities, such as those of the cells and tissues (Fig. 7).

Digestion begins in the mouth. Because food has been part of a living plant or animal, it carries a range of vibrations. Many of the subtler vibrations will be absorbed in the mouth and the finest are absorbed by the tongue. The longer the food remains in the mouth, the more benefit you will obtain – because this also allows the physical level of digestion to begin through the interaction of the saliva with the food.

EXERCISE 7: Blessing Your Food and Drink

Your physical nourishment has originally come from the Source, but it has taken form here on the planet. It is very beneficial to bless what you take into your body, to give thanks to the Source of food, to the planet, to the animals and plants which are being consumed and to those who have helped to bring it to your table. When food and drink are treated in this way, their spiritual energies are emphasized, subtle energies are raised, and cleared of any negativity. Furthermore, your attitude is so focused that the best conditions for digestion on all levels have been created.

○ Any formula which embraces all the above elements would be suitable, but best are the spontaneous words or thoughts of thanks which come at the time. Think about what you may like to do with your hands during this exercise.

The Breath and Breathing

The process of digestion is also enhanced by good breathing. Unless we suffer from a respiratory disorder such as asthma, we do not have to think about

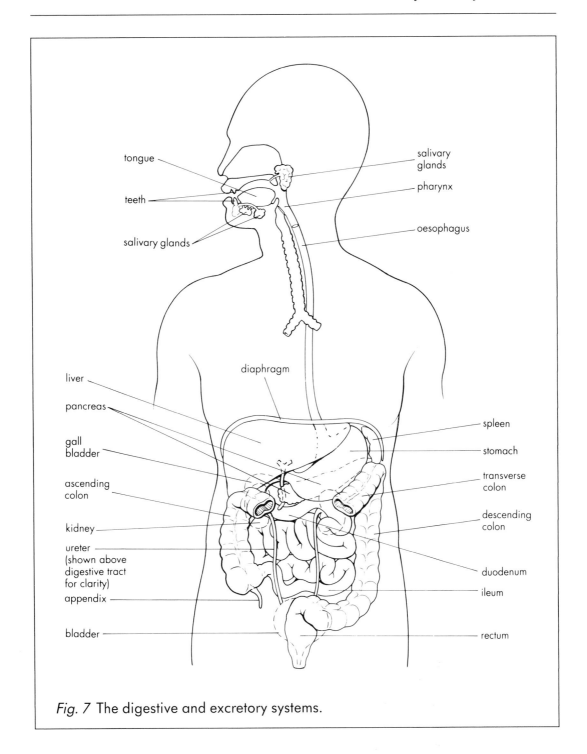

Fig. 7 The digestive and excretory systems.

breathing. Just like digestion and blood circulation, it is under the control of the autonomic nervous system. But we can intervene to control our breathing in a beneficial way. When we are upset, for example, the breathing rate speeds up which, in turn, increases heartbeat. By controlling the breath and calming it, we can regain our balance so that we are in a better state to cope.

Most people do not breathe properly and use only a small part of their lungs, often due to factors such as stress, bad posture and lack of exercise. We can change the bad habit of inefficient breathing by short, but regular, sessions of controlled breathing.

As well as vital oxygen, the life force (known as *prana* in Sanskrit) is present in air and partly enters our body through breathing. A knowledge of controlled breathing will allow you to enhance your intake of prana. Many of the exercises in this book involve the use of controlled breathing to enable you to interact more efficiently with healing energies.

EXERCISE 8: How Breathing Works

○ Sit comfortably and focus on your breathing. Notice what your body is doing while you breathe rhythmically and gently.

○ See if you can identify the parts of the body which are involved in the process.

Yes, the large muscle which forms the floor of your chest, the diaphragm, is doing most of the work (Fig. 8). When the diaphragm contracts downwards, the cavity enclosed by the rib cage is enlarged, creating a vacuum. The lungs are suspended in this cavity and expand to fill the space, automatically drawing in air via the nose or mouth. The diaphragm then expands by relaxing upwards, which deflates the lungs, thereby forcing the breath to be expired.

There are thus two breaths, the in-breath and the out-breath, both of which you may feel as different sensations. As air is breathed into the lungs, oxygen passes through their fine membranes into the bloodstream to oxygenate the cells and tissues. On the out-breath, waste gases such as carbon dioxide leave the bloodstream, to be expelled.

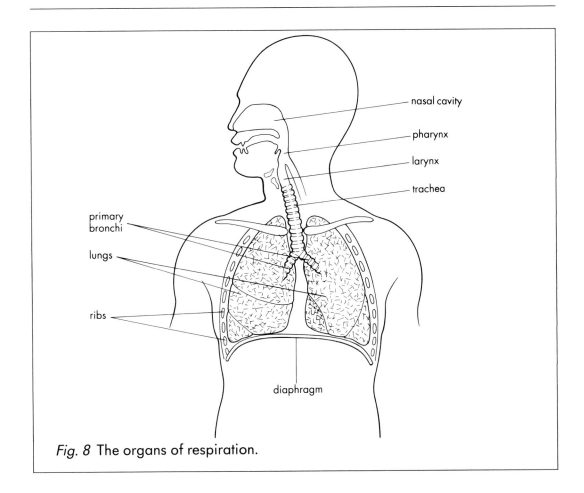

Fig. 8 The organs of respiration.

EXERCISE 9: Full Breath Breathing

This exercise should be taped or read out to you by a partner.

○ Sit comfortably with your feet flat on the floor. Notice your breathing. Allow it to become slow, deep and gentle.

○ Notice what your chest and abdomen are doing. Full breath breathing involves the movement of the abdomen. Put your hands there and imagine a balloon which is going to be filled and then totally emptied.

○ As you slowly inhale through the nose, allow the balloon to be filled by
  letting the abdomen gently swell outwards. Do not strain.

○ Breathe out as you feel the balloon of your abdomen deflate. Again, do
  not strain but empty slowly.

○ Do this exercise three times. Notice the difference between the in-breath
  and the out-breath. Notice how you feel as you breathe like this.

○ Now repeat with three more full breaths. This time hold the in-breath for
  a count of three.

○ Count three after the out-breath, before the next inhalation.

Full breath breathing aids digestion and sound sleep. Use it when you need to
calm down or think clearly. Use it when you feel depressed or unhappy. Use it
in the middle of a brisk walk if you have paused for a 'breather'.

The next time you see a baby or a small child asleep, notice the way s/he
breathes. How different is this to the way in which you breathe? The full breath
is also known as 'soft-belly breathing' because it encourages the relaxation of
the abdomen and discourages the tense, hard-belly approach to body posture.
Posture reflects our mood and attitude. It can also affect both in a positive way.
The soft-belly posture allows you to remain calm and balanced, to breathe more
deeply and maintain a centre of gravity below the navel.

The Nervous System

Most of the control and communication which goes on in the body is carried out
by the nervous system, which transmits its messages by means of electro-
chemical impulses, with the brain acting as the command centre. The
extensive network of nerves branching from the spinal cord, allows the brain to
keep in touch with all the other body systems and to process everything which
is happening to us internally and externally (Fig. 9).

The brain, with its convoluted covering of grey matter, the cortex, looks
something like a walnut. It is considered that the two halves or hemispheres of
the brain reflect our dual nature. The left hemisphere tends to deal with logical
thinking, analysis, mathematics, linear and verbal concepts. The right
hemisphere tends to deal with creative thinking, artistic, aesthetic, spatial,
non-linear and intuitive matters. People are sometimes described as 'right-' or

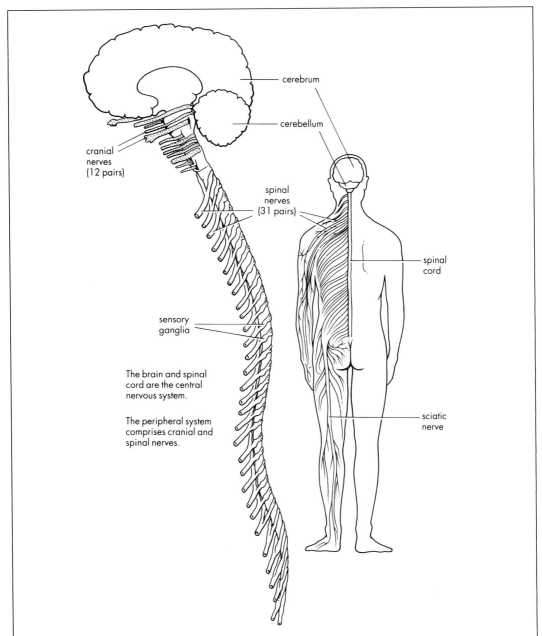

cerebrum

cerebellum

cranial
nerves
(12 pairs)

spinal
nerves
(31 pairs)

spinal
cord

sensory
ganglia

The brain and spinal
cord are the central
nervous system.

The peripheral system
comprises cranial and
spinal nerves.

sciatic
nerve

Fig. 9 The central nervous system, showing the brain, spinal cord, and spinal nerves. All other nerves are branches, or secondary and tertiary branches of the main structure.

'left-' brained, meaning that they seem to have such an emphasis to their personality. But the balanced development of both sides of the brain is necessary to obtain a holistic view of ourselves, those outside us and the universe in which we live.

The cerebral cortex is considered to be the most highly evolved area of the brain. It is concerned with storing experience and with the exchange and processing of nervous impulses. Most of the nerves which run to and from the cortex cross to the opposite side of the central nervous system. This means that, for example, the impulse to activate muscles on the left side of the body comes from the right side of the cortex, and vice versa.

Relaxation

The activity of the brain is slowed down when we are fully relaxed, creating the ideal state for meditation. This also applies to healing, where both patient and healer should be as relaxed as possible. Relaxation relieves tension and stress and allows our body energies to flow more freely. In the exercise which follows, you will send a command to the brain to allow all the muscles of the body to relax as much as possible. You will co-ordinate this with slow, deep and gentle breathing which immediately sends positive messages to all the body systems that things are becoming calm and peaceful. The benefits from this command to the brain are almost instantaneous.

EXERCISE 10: Full Body Relaxation

This exercise should be taped or read out to you by a partner.

○ Lie down with a support such as a pillow or small cushion beneath the head and neck.

○ Allow your legs to part and move your hands away from the sides of the body.

○ Carry out the full breath as in Exercise 9 (page 27). Breathe slowly, gently and normally.

○ Now focus on your hands. Clench them tightly then let them slowly unclench. Remember the feeling of unclenching (relaxing) and letting go.

Do not clench anything again throughout the rest of this exercise. As you breathe, know that you are breathing in peace and relaxation. Let any anxieties or problems go with the out-breath, breathe them out.

○ Now focus on the toes of your left foot. Feel them relax, one by one. Move slowly over your foot, relaxing the muscles. Let the ankle go.

○ Move up your left leg, relaxing the muscles. Let the knee joint go. Relax the big thigh muscles and the muscles of the buttocks.

○ Let go across the pelvis. Continue to breathe slowly and gently.

○ Focus on your right foot and proceed in the same way, over the foot and up the right leg, slowly and deliberately relaxing and letting go.

○ Relax the pelvis again.

○ Now come up the front of the body, relaxing the belly and stomach, letting go of the muscles of the chest. Let go of the shoulders.

○ Return to the lower back and slowly relax your back muscles, letting them go one by one. Pay particular attention to the muscles across the top of the back and shoulders – much tension gathers here. Relax and let go.

○ Relax the left shoulder and move down the left arm. Let the elbow joint go. Move down the forearm, relaxing and letting go. Let the wrist relax.

○ Relax the palm, fingers and thumb, one by one.

○ Return to the right shoulder. Relax it and move down the right arm in the same way. Relax the whole of the shoulder girdle.

○ Now move up your neck, very slowly, relaxing and letting go. Come up the back of the head and over the top of the scalp, relaxing and letting go of all the tiny muscles.

○ Imagine a caring hand smoothing your forehead. Relax the eyes, the cheeks, the mouth. Relax the jaw.

○ Continue to breathe slowly, gently and normally. Scan your body to see if any part has tensed up again. If it has, relax it, enjoying the feeling of total relaxation. You can remain mentally alert or allow yourself to drift off into sleep.

The next time you do this exercise, you might like to put on some quiet, soothing music. Practise relaxation so that it becomes second nature and you can do it anywhere, in any circumstances and in any position. When your body relaxes it has a beneficial knock-on effect on the other systems of the body, slowing down breathing and heartbeat, relieving stress and calming the mind. As well as being an essential requirement in all healing, relaxation *is* healing, for this act of letting go allows your energies to come back into balance.

The Endocrine System

The second of the body's two major control systems is the series of endocrine glands, the glands without ducts. The endocrine system transmits chemical messages in the form of hormones which are carried in the bloodstream.

When the word *hormone* originally came into use, around 1905, it had been derived from a Greek word meaning to urge on or excite. Since then it has been found that hormones can inhibit as well as stimulate body processes. They can slow down or speed up an activity, produce short or long-term effects, turn a process on or off. All these reactions are triggered by a feedback system which may be positive or negative so that, once the required effect has been produced, the endocrine system is continuously aware of the latest state of affairs and can modify any process.

The endocrine system and the numerous functions of its glands are very important to healers, for it is a system which has a special link with the etheric and other subtle levels of being. It not only carries out its physical functions, but receives and processes a range of subtle energies which have a direct effect on these functions. (The relationship between the endocrine system and the subtle energies is discussed in Chapter 4).

Starting at the bottom of Fig. 10, the **testes** in males control sexual development and maturity and the production of sperm.

The **ovaries** in females control sexual development and maturity and the production of eggs.

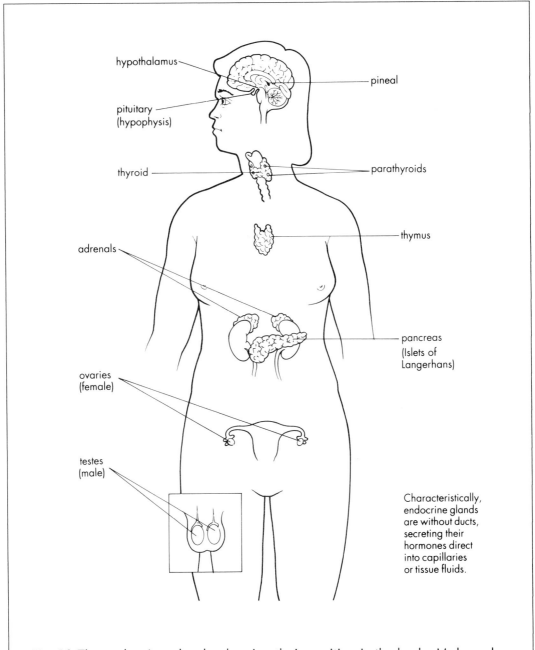

Fig. 10 The endocrine glands, showing their position in the body. Male and female glands are both illustrated.

Scattered throughout the pancreas are groups of endocrine cells, the **Islets of Langerhans**. These make a number of hormones, among which is insulin, the controller of the blood sugar level.

The **adrenal** glands, two glands in one, at the top of the kidneys, control the balance of salt in the body fluids and help prepare the body for emergencies through the secretion of adrenalin.

The **thymus** gland is closely related to the body's immune system. In childhood it controls the production of white blood cells, the 'T' lymphocytes which fight off infections and foreign bodies in the lymphatic system. It was thought that the activity of the thymus gland waned after puberty but recent research is beginning to question this.

The **thyroid** gland controls the rate of metabolism (use of fuel) and body growth. Embedded in the thyroid are the parathyroids which control the level of calcium in the blood.

The **hypothalamus** is the main controller of the **pituitary** gland and the endocrine system and monitors all information about body states. It is the main co-ordinator of the activities of the nervous and endocrine systems and acts as an intermediary between the body and the brain. The hypothalamus communicates with the pituitary either by nerve impulses or by its own hormones. These, in turn, stimulate the pituitary to secrete a range of hormones which have an effect on most of the body's functions, through the stimulation of other glands and organs (Fig. 10).

The **pineal** gland lies behind and above the hypothalamus. It is indirectly sensitive to light. As daylight fades to darkness, the pineal gland secretes the hormone melatonin. As daylight returns, secretion stops. During the winter months, melatonin secretion is higher than in summer. Thus, the pineal gland acts like a body clock and informs the body of the rhythm of day and night and the passing of the seasons.

This is the topmost gland of the endocrine system and, interestingly, it is affected by light and talks to the body about light. It is no coincidence that this gland is situated close to where spiritual light enters the body at a subtle level (Fig. 10).

KEEPING IN TOUCH WITH YOUR WHOLE BODY

Your body is your friend and the following exercises encourage you to be *in* and with your body, to take further steps in building the friendship.

EXERCISE 11: Being with the Body

○ Sit or lie comfortably. Relax and slow your breathing to settle to a gentle rhythm.

○ As you link with the rhythm of your breath, visualize that your body is gradually being surrounded with a golden light. You will find yourself becoming calm and serene as your awareness of the peaceful operations which are taking place within your body increases. This is your vehicle for your soul's expression on Earth. Your consciousness helped to make it what it is today. You dwell within this body of light wherein a million movements of energy are continually taking place. You can link up with the minutest part and the greatest part of this activity through the network of consciousness.

○ As you relax into the light which surrounds you, allow yourself to be.

This exercise can be continued for as long as you wish or you can move from this state to the next exercise.

EXERCISE 12: Sharing Body Secrets

Your body contains many secrets. Within its cells, it has stored memories about everything that has happened to it, from the time of conception until now.

○ Allow your attention to focus on a specific organ or part of your body and link up with it in your mind. Allow this part of your body to show you what it has stored. Accept what comes. It may be in the form of words, pictures, or sensations.

EXERCISE 13: Energy through the Skin

From Exercise 12 you can move to the perception of energy flow through the skin.

○ Focus on your skin as an envelope of awareness, keeping you in touch with the energies around you. Allow yourself to be aware of the energies which surround you at the moment.

○ As you relax more and more into your awareness, see if you can distinguish different energies. Are there any you do not like or which make you feel uncomfortable?

○ Allow yourself to become aware of the energies of peace and love which flow all around you. Sink into them and feel the flow of them. They are absorbed into your skin through the pores and penetrate all your organs and every cell of your body. See this beneficial system flowing freely, carrying the force of life within you.

Try this exercise out of doors, standing, sitting or lying down. How did it differ when you did the exercise outside? Note any patterns or structures you see in your mind's eye as you spend time with the exercise.

In the exercises of being with the body, try to resist analysis at least until the communication has finished. If you are ill or have suffered an injury, listen to what your body may have to tell you about it. If you locate a certain mood or feeling somewhere in your body, allow these parts of yourself to talk to you about your perceptions and sensations.

When communication has finished, in your mind's eye see the golden glow of energy around you change to pink, the colour of love. Let this pink energy penetrate every part of your body. Give it your thanks.

By the time you have concluded the body exercises you may be in a state which is close to meditation. Make sure you can feel your feet. Wiggle your toes. Make sure you have returned to a 'normal' state before you get up and carry on with other things. Perhaps, like William Blake, you now feel that your body is not as distinct from your soul as you first thought!

2

Bodies of Light –
The Subtle Bodies

*J*ohn asked me to accompany him to the hospice where his mother was dying. It was a bad time for John. Other things were going wrong in his life and he didn't need the added strain of his mother's terminal illness – he needed support. I said I would do my best to help.

We found his mother sitting up in bed. The tan of her skin, due to the treatment she was receiving, gave her the appearance of being well. But her arms were swollen with the cancer which had spread throughout her body. While she and John talked together I held her hand, and soon she dropped off to sleep. The breath rattled in her throat as she slept peacefully.

I thought I had dropped off too, for suddenly I seemed to be dreaming, seeing two mothers. One was asleep while the other leaned forward and smiled at us. She looked radiant, surrounded by a faint glow of light. She seemed younger and slimmer too. I was aware of her words or thoughts in my mind. Though her lips were not moving, she was talking to John, reassuring him. Then she slipped out of the bed and glided from the room. I could see John was aware of what was happening too, for he looked at his 'other' mother who was still asleep with me holding her hand.

He then looked at me with tears in his eyes. 'Did you see that?' he whispered.

I nodded.

'She's going to be all right.'

It was a statement about his own conviction. He visibly relaxed and began to smile broadly.

On the way back from the hospice, John seemed unable to contain his excitement. He told me how his mother had spoken to him in a very special way, showing him his life problems in a new and more positive light, as if she had disentangled them before his eyes. 'It all happened in a second. I felt so happy, wondering why I couldn't feel sad about Mum. I still don't feel sad . . .'

The next day John's mother died peacefully in her sleep.

LEVELS OF BEING: THE SUBTLE BODIES

Your response to John's experience will indicate your degree of readiness to accept the concept of human subtle anatomy. Perhaps you have had a similar experience or know someone who has. The next two chapters will help you understand such experiences, how and why things like this happen.

John's mother was in a different body when she walked out of the terminal ward where her physical body was in the process of dying. When I feel and see the bodies of people during a distant healing session, they are not physical bodies either. These bodies, though not at all wraithlike or fragile, are composed of finer material which gives them the impression of being bodies of light. In both instances, they are what is known as the *etheric* body, one of a number of subtle bodies which, along with the physical body, go to make the whole human being.

The Etheric Body

Being the closest to the physical, this is the first of the subtle bodies which may be sensed. To those who are able to see it, it looks like a misty material projecting an inch or two beyond the physical or it may be felt, especially with your hands. It is composed of matter vibrating at speeds just above the velocity of light, which makes it invisible to our everyday senses. We all possess high sense perception at different degrees of development and it is this faculty which allows us to sense energies beyond those vibrating at the physical level. High sense perception can be developed by training and many of the exercises in this book will help you to do this. All matter is energy and it is the quality of this energy which your brain interprets as colour, feeling, sound, and so on.

This second body of ours came to be called the *etheric* body, from the ancient Greek term which referred to the upper regions of the atmosphere or heaven as *ether*. Seers of the time had witnessed that, on passing over, people carried on being in their 'heavenly' or etheric body.

This is the body which John saw and with which healers often work during healing. From the point of view of healing, it is perhaps the most important body and one which you will get to know very well by the time you have completed more of the exercises.

The etheric body has been known to many cultures since ancient times. The seers of India and China have described it in detail, making diagrams to illustrate their findings. Other aboriginal cultures such as the Native American, Polynesian and Australian were aware of the etheric energy system and this has been codified within their art, music, costume and oral traditions.

In spite of this evidence, the presence of an energy field around living things was discounted by science because it could not be detected by current technology. Then, in the 1890s, a Polish nobleman, Yakub Yodko-Narkevitch, began investigating a form of photography which used a high voltage, high frequency electric charge instead of light. This enabled him to 'photograph' the energy emanations given off by living material.

With the Russian Revolution his findings were lost until the technique was rediscovered accidentally by Semyon Kirlian in 1939. A similar charge was passed across a film on which certain biological specimens had been placed and strange light patterns were found to occur around these specimens. No light source was used and yet a corona of energy showed up each time.

Corona-discharge photography (also known as Kirlian photography) was classified as secret by the Soviet government until 1960, when Kirlian published a report with his wife, Valentina. In it, the corona discharge image was claimed to be the scientific evidence of a bio-energy field. Their report created tremendous interest in scientific circles worldwide. Clairvoyants saw it as proof of what they had always been perceiving through high sense perception.

Researchers in other parts of the world went on to discover that the light given out by a subject varied according to the vital or living force present. For example, a leaf plucked straight from a tree showed an energy field which grew smaller as the leaf dried out. The corona around a healthy leaf was markedly different to that around leaves taken from infected plants. Not surprisingly, photographs of healers' hands showed a significant increase in the energy discharge when healing was being given.

Kirlian photography has shown that there seems to be an invisible matrix or energy blueprint at the bio-energy level from which every living thing develops. Photographs of leaf sections, for example, always show the full outline of the leaf before it was cut. This is known as the 'phantom leaf' effect (Fig. 11). Photographs of hands with missing fingers also show the energy matrix as complete, supporting the findings of clairvoyants and healers that there is a complete blueprint of the physical body present at the etheric level.

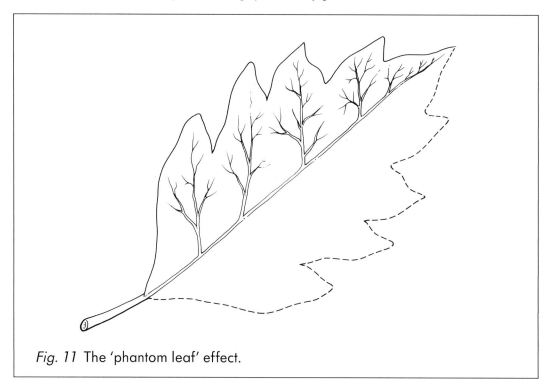

Fig. 11 The 'phantom leaf' effect.

The etheric level acts as a 'bridge' between two very different levels of being – the physical and the subtle levels. As we shall see in the next chapter, part of this function is to act as the preparation level for entry into the Earth plane. So souls who have decided to experience the Earth plane will first have to acquire an etheric body.

A second and equally important function of the etheric body relates to its actual form. Within it are structures which allow us to absorb high frequency energies, including the vital or life force, which are processed at the etheric level before being passed on into the physical body. These energetic structures of the etheric body, the *chakras*, will be discussed in Chapter 4.

The Astral Body

The body which appears to project beyond the etheric is in the next higher frequency range, the astral. Because its vibrations are finer than the etheric, we can travel at will in this body with even less limitation, by the power of thought. At the astral level of vibration, the energies of feeling are processed. This is why some authorities call the astral body the *emotional* body. At higher astral levels, the higher emotions related to unconditional love, such as compassion and empathy, are processed. At lower astral levels, fear and the more negative emotions are processed ('lower' in this context refers to a denser frequency range of matter).

We all enter the astral levels during the sleep state. Here, we can meet up with other souls or travel to places which we would have difficulty in reaching in our everyday life. Some healers do a great deal of their work in their astral bodies, during sleep and waking states. This accounts for reports of healers appearing in their patients' homes at all times of the day or night and also appearing to them in their dreams.

We also go into our astral body to receive teaching, instructions and initiation during the sleep state. Do not be surprised if you start having dreams like this once you begin working with the book! Record all such experiences in your journal and spend some time considering what your adventures on the astral are saying to you.

The Mental Bodies

The next frequency range which can be detected is what is known as the mental level. On this higher frequency than the astral, the mental bodies process a range of mental energies, including creative and intuitive thought. Those who can sense the energies of the mental bodies find that they extend beyond the astral.

The Soul Body

Finally, the soul itself is enclosed in a containment vehicle or body, in order to go through the whole human experience, and this is vibrating at frequencies far beyond the levels already mentioned. All experience at all levels is conveyed back to the soul – the real you – through the network of consciousness.

THE HUMAN ENERGY FIELD OR AURA

At this point you may have a picture of yourself as something like a set of Russian dolls, of bodies within bodies. The important difference is that the individual rate of vibration of the various bodies allows them to be inter-penetrating rather than simply one inside the other. You have a number of bodies but you are only aware of them when you are conscious of their relevant levels of experience. Each body is a specific pattern which radiates energy, like the bars of an electric fire. The emanation of each body gives it a glowing luminosity which varies in intensity from person to person. To those with developed high sense perception the combined effect of all the interpenetrating bodies is like a multi-coloured aura of light around the physical body. This is the human energy field or aura (Fig. 12).

Interpreting the Aura

Writers differ in their interpretation of the aura. This is partly due to their own experience and partly due to the extent of their knowledge. You will find it useful to go by your own experience as far as possible and to build on this. What you can see and sense depends on your own level of spirituality and your developed high sense perception.

The energetic structure of the aura contains information about the current state of a person's body, mind, emotions and spiritual development. It also contains a record of every experience undergone by the soul. This is why the aura is so important in healing.

Sceptics may think that it is not possible to sense this total energy field, to discriminate between the different levels and to interpret the material that they contain. But there are many healers in practice for whom this is a regular aspect of their work. Such awareness is available to all through training, enhanced personal development and increased sensitivity.

Whatever level the soul has experienced will be present as energy within the aura. Individual souls vary in their experience and their development so each human aura is unique.

The soul is able to experience some levels without acquiring a vehicle (or body), but its experience on these levels will still be registered in an individual's energy field.

Most people on the planet at this time will be emanating the energy levels shown in Fig. 12. But certain people on the planet emanate auras which contain energies not confined to bodies alone. There are highly-evolved children, for example, who have these.

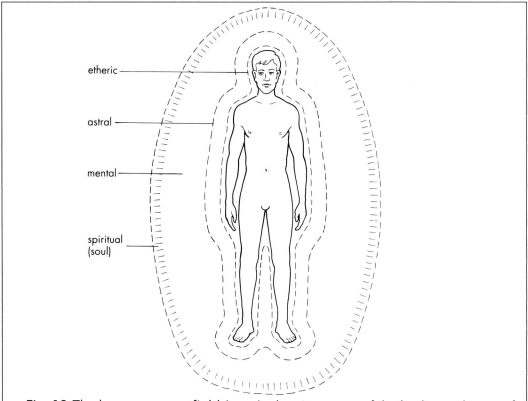

Fig. 12 The human energy field (aura), showing some of the bodies or layers of experience which can be sensed through developed high sense perception.

With practice, you will find that you can sense the energies of the physical aura. After a time you may be able to experience and identify the finer vibrations of the etheric and astral levels. These vibrations are then interpreted by the brain as colours or other impressions. When you find you are able to *experience* an energy field as knowledge, rather than impressions, you will be sensing at a spiritual level.

The greatest part of the aura, though rarely sensed by others, is the emanation of the soul or inner Self. The Self is a reflection of the Source and the extent of its emanation indicates the extent of a person's development. Just as the evolving Self is constantly changing through the experiences it undergoes, so the level of its development changes as lessons are learned and consciousness expands. All such changes are registered in the aura as changes of energy flow and energy quality. So the aura is the energy record of our total being at any moment in time.

The Aura as a Diagnostic Aid

When Maureen came for healing she was obviously anxious about something. She was not used to talking too much about her problems so we got straight on with the healing session. After attuning with her I began by scanning her aura. It projected further on one side of her body than the other where it felt quite weak. There was a grey cloud around her head and this grey colour occurred again in her solar plexus region.

When I had completed the hands-on healing, I told Maureen what I had noticed in her aura. It indicated that she was worrying a great deal and feeling upset about someone. This someone was close to her, which made her aura project out more on one side than the other. She was so surprised, that she began to talk about her husband who had been ill for some time. She was a born worrier, she said, and she was also worried about becoming ill herself. She was able to express feelings which she had at first decided were better kept repressed.

So the aura scan not only picked up Maureen's emotional state, but also the root cause of her condition. The healing helped to balance her and she enjoyed some practice at slow and gentle breathing to calm her mind. At the next session, the scan revealed that Maureen's system had started to balance itself. The grey cloud around her head had diminished and her aura was more regular in shape.

STARTING TO WORK WITH AURAS

Experiences like this broaden and enhance the information which a patient may or may not have already volunteered. With practice, you will develop your own ways of receiving data from another person's aura. This helps to build up a more comprehensive view of them and, in cases like Maureen's, provides a valuable starting point for helping someone to express his or her feelings.

Here are two important exercises to get you working with auras and enjoying the feeling of sensitivity which you will become aware of. You will need a partner to work with. In each case, remind yourself that you are sensing the light of another person. Honour this as a special gift from them to you.

EXERCISE 14: Sensing the Aura

○ Ask your partner to stand, with feet slightly apart (Fig. 13a), to relax and breathe normally.

○ Stand in front of your partner and hold the palms of your hands a body's width away from your partner's head. Slowly bring your palms in towards the head until you feel a change in the energy between your hand and your partner's head. (When your sensitivity has developed sufficiently you will be able to feel the energy radiating from the head as you 'bounce' your palms gently against this field.)

○ Now slowly bring your palms down the body, continuing to trace the energy field around it. Notice how far from the body it seems to project. Be prepared for it to change. Does it swell out or go in at any point?

○ Repeat the process down the front and back of your partner's body. How far above the top of the head does it extend?

○ Next, to find out if the field seems to extend from the feet also, ask your partner to lie down and see what the emanations are from the feet.

You have now built up a picture of the total energy field which surrounds your partner. As you do the exercise, you might pick up colours, an unusual shape to the energy field or variations in temperature. These are all part of your interpretation of your partner's energy field. See if your partner can relate to your findings.

This exercise should be repeated from time to time. One experience of sensing another's aura will not teach you all there is to know. See if you become aware of 'layers' in the aura. Make a note of how you were aware of this. Some people experience the energies of an aura as areas of heat or coldness. If this happens to you, decide what you think this means in terms of your partner's health and general balance of energy. Discuss these findings with your partner.

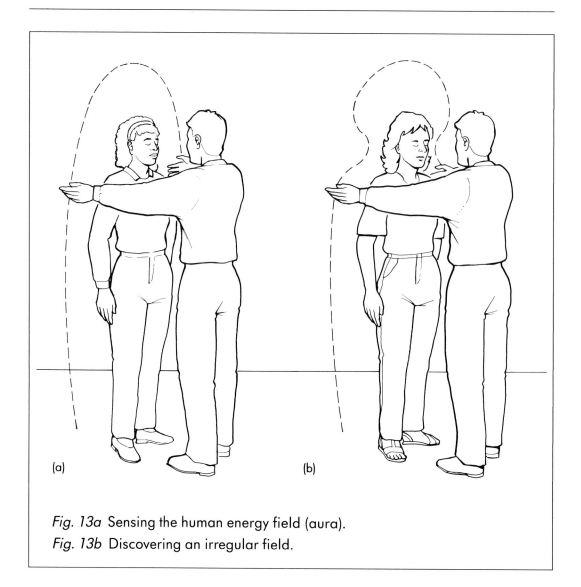

(a)   (b)

Fig. 13a Sensing the human energy field (aura).
Fig. 13b Discovering an irregular field.

EXERCISE 15: Illustrating Your Perceptions

○ Now try to illustrate your experience, using colours where necessary. Show your partner your illustration. Can your partner interpret it?

EXERCISE 16: Impressions from a Partner's Aura

○ Sit opposite a new partner. Close your eyes. Relax as much as possible and let your breathing become slow and rhythmic.

○ Allow your attention to focus on the energy field surrounding your partner. At the same time your partner should focus on your energy field. Wait patiently for impressions to flow into your consciousness.

○ Do not be judgmental or analytical, but try to accept exactly what comes. Make a note of what impressions you receive about your partner. Your partner should do the same about you.

○ Discuss your impressions and ask your partner to comment. When you assess all the impressions which you have both received from each other, what do you think are the implications of this? How do you think it is possible to receive such information from someone else without a word being spoken and without body language or facial signals being taken into account?

This exercise is most effective with someone you have never met before. Your impressions may include their temperament, current mood, state of health, things that have happened to them, other people in their life, and so on. You may also receive impressions as symbols, colours, feelings and thoughts. There may be an indication of a problem or worry.

During a recent workshop where people were asked to sense the aura, a woman found her partner's aura suddenly 'going in' in the region of the jaw (see Fig. 13b). When she asked about it, her partner said she had been recently suffering from a bad toothache.

At the same workshop, a man was surprised to sense the energy of his partner's aura as warmth. He was further surprised to find that this stopped when his scan was on a level with the knees. Then he felt the aura become cold. His partner was surprised that the scan had revealed that he had very poor circulation and varicose veins in the lower legs.

In both of these cases you may have sensed these conditions in another way. Go by your own impressions and be prepared to trust them, for this is how it is possible to access such important information from working with the aura alone.

'You think of us as beings of light and joy, which we are, but you seldom think of humans as beings of light, which you are.'

THE ANGEL OF FENNEL
Dorothy Maclean

3

Your Soul Journey

Working with patients has taught me that everyone is on a journey. Everybody's journey is unique and some travel fast, some slow, some travel light, some bring along plenty of baggage, but we are all heading for the same destination. My way may be different to yours but we're sure to meet up sometime.

You have an aura, which is an emanation of all the subtle bodies, because you came on a soul journey, a journey through realms of light. By taking a brief look at what happens on the journey you will be able to understand how you came to have subtle bodies as well as a physical one and why spiritual healing addresses itself to all these aspects of your being and not just the physical alone.

THE PATHS OF INVOLUTION AND EVOLUTION

From the Source of all that is, known as God, outpourings of energy were projected. The interaction of these energies brought about the creation of matter, the different levels of experience with their different universes. Into this creation the human soul or divine spark was projected on a journey of experience, learning and expression. During the first phase of the journey we have moved down through levels of being to the physical or Earth plane. This is the path of involution. From this level we are making our journey back – the path of evolution (Fig. 14). Every experience that we have is instantly known to the Source through the network of consciousness.

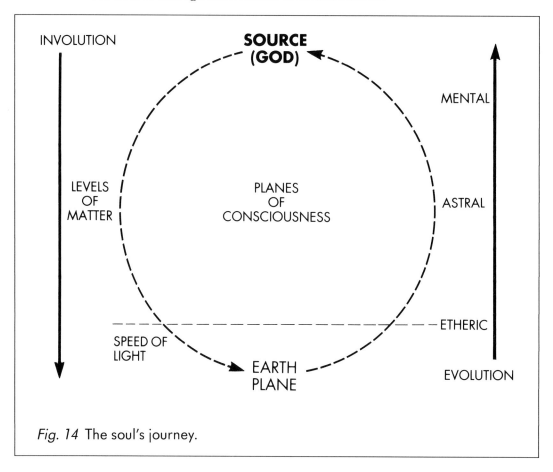

INVOLUTION

SOURCE
(GOD)

MENTAL

LEVELS
OF
MATTER

PLANES
OF
CONSCIOUSNESS

ASTRAL

SPEED OF
LIGHT

ETHERIC

EARTH
PLANE

EVOLUTION

Fig. 14 The soul's journey.

This is a bare outline of your journey. The real story is about the adventures you have had on your way, and those that are still to come. Your story began when you left home, the Source. Here on Earth you may feel very far from home, perhaps facing your greatest challenge.

As soon as the soul enters the physical level, it becomes aware of a sense of separation which is further emphasized by the limitations of the physical body. In this way, the Earth plane provides unique learning situations for the soul. The apparent separation from other people and other forms of life, for example, encourages us to develop a separate personality (the ego). We tend to identify with this and it soon becomes easy to assume that our personality is all we are.

Healers have found that the personality's experience of separation and limitation is the cause of many of the difficulties which people encounter, from childhood onwards.

But before you got here you already had experience and encounters on the subtle levels of being. Now, these experiences radiate from you, as the energies of your aura. Some may see their beautiful colours, others their pictures, still others may sense them in ways difficult to describe. This total spiritual being is what healing works with. Healers talk about applying healing energies to body, mind and spirit. What they mean by 'spirit' is the journeying soul.

CHALLENGING THE LIMITS OF CONDITIONING

Whereas in the past the subtle levels (those outside of the physical) were relegated to the realms of esoteric mystery, quantum physics and mathematics have made discoveries which have opened the way for science to consider the implications of what many clairvoyants and many healers know and experience. Since Einstein exploded Newtonian concepts about the nature of matter it could be said that physics has once more joined hands with metaphysics, waiting for religion to catch up.

Before Einstein's theories of relativity, physicists could not conceive of anything existing at velocities beyond the speed of light. Modern researchers, such as William Tiller, have further extended his theories to consider this concept. It seems that, if the velocity of matter continued to accelerate, a point would be arrived at where energy would reach infinite proportions. Spiritual healers would say that this would be the same source of infinite energy described by mystics and given various names by religion (referred to in this book as the Source).

Confronting this issue is difficult for many people because we have been thoroughly conditioned to regard life from the physical aspect alone. By working with this book you can challenge the limitations of your conditioning and see your life from a broader and freer perspective. The exercises will help develop your high sense perception so that you can become aware of what you are as a total being and acknowledge your human structure. This structure of light, with all its various energy patterns, is you. Gradually, awareness about yourself will show you that other people too are unique patterns of light.

The following exercises, like Exercise 1 in Chapter 1, are about getting used to the idea of being an energy pattern, a pattern of living light. To carry them out effectively, you will need to be as relaxed as possible and trust your awareness and your feelings.

EXERCISE 17: Looking for the Light Within

○ Sit with your feet flat on the ground, the hands resting on the thighs, elbows relaxed. Take three deep breaths then breathe normally.

○ Now look down at your hands. They appear solid. Realizing that this is the way you perceive and interpret their energy, imagine that the skin encloses shining light.

○ As your body relaxes, scan slowly up your arms and around your body, visualizing the light beneath the skin. How do you feel? Make a note of that and whatever else you notice.

EXERCISE 18: Breathing the Light

○ Notice your breathing, as you breathe quite normally. You breathe in and out through your nose. You are aware of your nose and your lungs especially.

○ Now close your eyes and visualize white light all around you. Focus on the light in front of you.

○ As you breathe in, imagine you can breathe this light into your face, then into the front of your body and your arms, then into your abdomen, then into your pelvis and legs.

○ Make a note of what you were aware of this time.

EXERCISE 19: Being Light

○ Every day for a week, visualize that you are a being filled with white light. You are a unique pattern of light moving among other patterns of light.

○ How did this affect your perception of yourself? How did it affect your perception of other people? How did others react to you? Did it affect your awareness of the world around you?

○ Make a note of these and other effects you experienced.

Each time you do the exercises you will be aware of different things, so it is worth repeating them. With practice, you will become more aware of the energy which is within and all around you and which surrounds others and is part of them. This link of energy, originating from the one Source, is what makes us one with each other and with all things. Life is the infinite expression of this oneness.

EXPLORING THE LEVELS OF CONSCIOUSNESS

To experience the different levels of being, the soul becomes embodied. The embodied soul is referred to in this book as the Self or Higher Self. This is who you are, the real you. As was explained in Chapter 2, on certain levels you need a body which is compatible with its surroundings – which vibrates at the same rate. For without the limitations of a body, you could pass through any vibration of matter without experiencing it.

To give an illustration, imagine that you are composed of such fine energies that, on a certain level, you can simply pass through the coarser energies of a wall or door. If, however, you surround yourself with a body which is vibrating at about the same rate as the wall or door, you can no longer pass through them. If this body has a consciousness with which you can link, you will be able to experience what it is like to be on that level. The levels are thus levels of consciousness.

In this way, you, the journeying soul, acquire all the bodies you need to travel on the levels of being you wish to explore. The layers or bodies which you may detect in someone's aura are actually the energetic record of their experience on these various levels.

On your journey to the Earth plane, before you reach the astral levels you will have experienced different spiritual and mental states. On the astral you still have great freedom of movement and here you experience different states of feeling and emotion, ranging from unconditional love to fear.

THE ETHERIC BLUEPRINT

You decided to come to the Earth plane as part of your evolutionary journey so you will have acquired an etheric body also. This preparation level is essential because of the dramatic differences between the astral and the physical, the differences between a state of astral being and the space/time dimensions of the Earth plane. The etheric level thus acts as a bridge between them, a place where the soul can prepare for the change in being which it will encounter. On the etheric level the design and creation of the physical body takes place. Here is formed the template or etheric blueprint from which the structure of the human body will be generated. The specific etheric matrix for each baby is in turn a modification of the general one.

There are many studies which show that the development of the etheric matrix precedes the development of actual physical forms. For example, in Geoffrey Hodson's *The Miracle of Birth: A Clairvoyant Study of a Human Embryo* he noted that soon after conception an etheric form appeared which resembled a baby body built of etheric matter composed of lines of force. The projection of the lines of force, he observed, influenced the laying down of the baby's physical body.

Professor Kim Bong Han, researching in Korea in the 1960s, found that the etheric meridian system of a chick was detectable within fifteen hours of conception, before the formation of rudimentary body organs. This confirms esoteric findings that the *etheric* body has to be in place before the laying down of the physical body.

At the physical level, of course, the building of the body from the blueprint is also subject to genetic and other physical factors and is under the control of the baby's mother. (The role of healing in birth and the entry of a new soul onto the Earth plane will be looked at in more detail in Chapter 14.)

HEALING AND YOUR SOUL JOURNEY

Throughout your life you absorb, interact with and generate energies on all the different levels of experience to which you are connected. For much of the time you are only conscious of your physical experiences. This is a kind of safety valve which ensures that you do not get distressed or confused through having to deal with more than one level of psychological material at a time.

The process begins at the subtler levels and the energies are passed through the series of bodies until they reach the etheric. Any emotional or mental disturbance you have experienced in life will create blocks to this flow which are registered in your etheric body. This will then influence the energies of the physical and have a direct bearing on your health.

Perhaps the most important implication of this process is that, by the time some complaint is registering in your physical, things have already gone awry on the subtler levels of being. So it is to here that healing will first be directed.

Each soul is unique and each of us comes to Earth with a mission to carry out. As well as working with dis-ease and imbalance, healers are involved in helping people achieve their mission and align the wants of the personality with the needs of the Higher Self. This means that whatever the condition presented, the healer will be addressing the spiritual aspects of a patient as well as the personality. Because we are dealing with souls, the healing link is made with the Higher Self of a person, with the confidence that the Higher Self will know how to make the best use of the energies for the presented condition and for those conditions which may not be presented.

Some people will need to understand if their condition is furthering their journey or perhaps interrupting or undermining it. Spiritual healing brings clarity to those who are struggling with dilemmas like these. At the same time it works in a gentle yet powerful way to change attitudes, to awaken insight and to bring the strength and peace of acceptance, as well as to help with the condition.

A soul has a threefold purpose in being on any level and that is to experience, to learn and to express itself. People seek healing as part of their journey and the condition they present will be reflecting one or more of these aspects. So illness may be a necessary part of someone's experience, their learning or even their self-expression. Equally, some need to realize that good health is a necessary part of their experience and not the conditions of ill health they are putting themselves through. The personality may find it difficult to accept, but these things are for the purpose of the soul.

4

The Chakras

*S*tan *clung to the edge of the iron cage. Outside the pithead, machines clanked and clattered, engines roared and steamed. He held his breath as long as he could, but the cold, damp, dust-laden air seemed to seep into his lungs and form a film over his skin. The men were laughing and joking. He could smell them and he could smell his own fear. He wanted to be sick. Suddenly an old miner looked him in the eyes and touched his arm. 'You'll be all right, butt.' Stan fought back the tears. It was his first shift. He was 14.*

Over 50 years later, Stan could recall the scene as he sat having healing. He had been a miner all his life until he was invalided out of the colliery. He had not liked his job, but in his village it had been the only work available. He contracted diabetes, which later threatened to affect his legs in the form of gangrene.

During the course of healing treatment, a powerful block was discovered in Stan's solar plexus chakra. This could be traced to his early days in the mines. He dreaded each shift and his stomach rose into his mouth every time the pit cage dropped to take him to his work at the coal face. Though he had got through each day bravely, his fear and anxiety never left him. He was only able to cope through the friendship of his mates and the support of people in the community.

Stand needed help to clear the energy block, to heal it and come to terms with his real and imagined fears. He was also given exercises in relaxation and stress release to back up the healing. One of the important benefits of the treatment was that Stan learned how to get in touch with his feelings and to express them to his wife and his friends.

STORING NEGATIVE ENERGY IN THE CHAKRAS

Stan's energy system had probably never been in a state of balance. His case illustrates the fact that, as well as storing negative energy in the weakest parts of the physical body, such as a hip, we store it in the chakras – the main energy centres of the etheric system. Here it may have an even more destructive effect for, apart from causing problems in the surrounding physical organs, it blocks the flow of energies which is so vital to our total wellbeing.

This occurs because, as Stan's case shows, things that happen to us in life can enhance or inhibit the flow of subtle energy. When unpleasant or disturbing things present themselves we try to avoid dealing with the issue in an attempt to minimize their impact upon us. This means that we do not fully process the energies involved and instead they have to be stored in the subtle bodies, especially in the chakras.

In this way, everything that happens on the emotional and mental levels has an energetic impact on the etheric body. This in turn impacts on the physical. Most of us are only aware of a change at the physical level and have no idea that this may be the symptom of a cause within the subtle bodies.

If the process of storing negative energies in a chakra continues without attention, it accumulates and the function of the chakra becomes impaired. Ultimately a chakra can become blocked and virtually ceases to function. This has a progressive effect throughout the system, with other chakras attempting to compensate for the inactive or blocked centre. Additional strain is then produced elsewhere in the energy system.

These effects may manifest as emotional or mental problems or a physical condition. Because the system always seeks to balance itself, to bring us to a state of harmony, it sends signals to us to draw our attention to the problem. On the physical level this is usually in the form of pain or the beginnings of some state of dis-ease.

The chakras are focal points for the energies of the subtle bodies where stored energy patterns can be accessed. This is why the study of the etheric body is so important for healers and why the chakras are the key to restoring balance.

GATEWAYS INTO THE ETHERIC BODY

It is helpful, then, to think of the chakras as gateways into the etheric body. There are some 360 of them, occurring at strategic positions related to the energetic functioning of the etheric and physical bodies. They range in size and function, from the seven major chakras aligned with the physical spine, to those situated in the palms of the hands, soles of the feet, behind the knees, at the elbows, and the minor ones scattered throughout the body.

The Sanskrit word *chakra*, now in common usage, comes from the ancient Indian tradition where healers and teachers with well-developed high sense perception identified them in the etheric body as whirling vortices of energy.

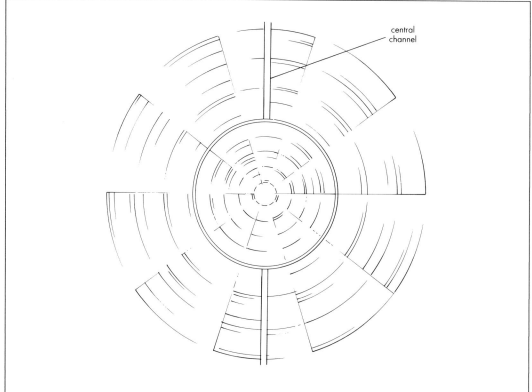

central
channel

Fig. 15 A major chakra. Front view showing nadis radiating from the central energy vortex.

They appeared to resemble cartwheels, an impression given by the smaller channels (*nadis*) which radiate from the centre of each chakra, so they were called *chakras* – wheels (Fig. 15).

There are many descriptions of the chakras, but what matters most is your experience of them. Learn how to sense where they are and what they are doing. A common image is of a funnel-shaped structure, somewhat like a convolvulus flower. When working with clients I have been able to see the structure of certain chakras. I have also witnessed the reconstruction of a throat chakra, illustrated in below.

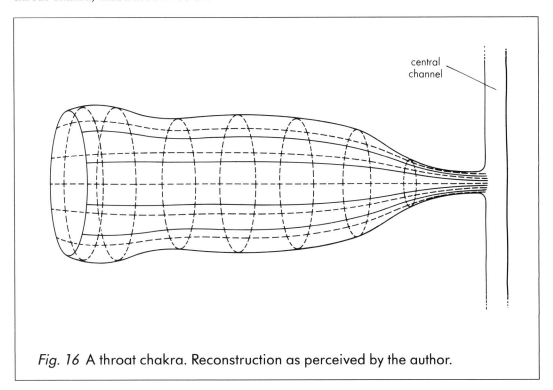

central
channel

Fig. 16 A throat chakra. Reconstruction as perceived by the author.

The lines in the figure should be imagined as lines of pale blue light. During the reconstruction, a grid-like pattern was first formed which gave the chakra its basic tubular shape. Finer lines were then wound round and round the grid, like thread, until the spaces were filled. The completed structure appeared luminous, strong yet delicate. This description is offered for you to compare with your own perceptions.

THE MERIDIANS

The chakras are linked by a system of fine etheric channels which are closely aligned to the nervous and vascular systems of the physical body. This fine etheric network provides the basis of the meridian system known to acupuncture.

The **meridian system** was first documented in China some 4000 years ago in *The Yellow Emperor's Classic of Internal Medicine*. It was discovered that the meridians conveyed the life force, *qi*, and that if the network became blocked it prevented the proper flow of the life force. The network radiates out from the chakras and main organs at a deep level to pass very close to the surface of the skin. Here the points of interconnection (acupuncture points) are located.

Modern research has found that the acupuncture points show a characteristically low electrical resistance. This demonstrates that these points in the etheric network are places where energy becomes concentrated because of the interconnection of two or more fine channels.

Studies in the 1960s by Korean researchers, and later by French researchers, have confirmed the presence of the network in an interesting way. The fine etheric channels were found to convey organic nutrients in solution which were directly assimilated by the body cells. This provides the physical means whereby the life force, first entering the system via the breath and bloodstream, can be carried in solution to every cell of the body, where it is transmitted to the nucleus.

The life force stimulates the nucleus to carry out and oversee cell activities. If it does not reach the nucleus, cell activities cease and the body begins the process of disintegration.

THE MULTIPLE FUNCTIONS OF THE CHAKRAS

Thus, one of the important functions of the chakra network is to convey the life force to the nucleus of every cell in the body. Each chakra also facilitates the flow and interchange of energies from the subtle levels by stepping them down, so that they can be used by the physical body. Similarly, the frequency of energies can be stepped up so that they can be utilized at the subtle levels. They also allow for the input and output of energies *through* the centres.

The seven major chakras are points of energy entry into and exit from different levels of consciousness as well as providing the connecting links between these levels.

FOUR OTHER CHAKRAS IMPORTANT IN HEALING

Two pairs of chakras should also be noted – those in the palms of the hands and those in the soles of the feet. Like all chakras, they are transmitters and absorbers of energy.

The **palm** chakras are able to transmit healing energies. Homeopathic remedies, flower and gem essences should never be held in the palm of the hand because their energy pattern is immediately absorbed by the palm chakra.

The chakras in the **soles of the feet** absorb energy from the planet, the ground beneath our feet. They are involved in earthing or grounding certain of the body energies and in helping to create a complete circuit for healing energies. This is why both healer and patient need to be aware of this connection at the start of a healing session. This connection should also be emphasized at the start of meditation or any other spiritual exercise.

THE CHAKRAS ARE UNIVERSAL

The ancient Indians preferred to use a single concept word for such multifunctional structures rather than a number of phrases which would define them in a more limited way.

The English names of the chakras reflect their relative position in the body, but it is worth studying the ancient concepts about them for this will broaden your knowledge. Knowledge about the chakras has not been confined to the Orient, as is often thought, and they are certainly not part of any particular belief system or religion. They are known to many other ancient cultures.

It is interesting to note, for example, how Native American nations have used jewellery and decoration to protect or stimulate specific energy centres.

In the West, where a great deal of esoteric knowledge has been suppressed, coded references survive such as those in *The Revelation of St. John The Divine* in the *New Testament* of *The Bible*. Here the 'seven churches' of Asia, which feature prominently in the early chapters, are thought by some scholars to refer to the seven chakras.

THE SEVEN MAJOR CHAKRAS

Moving in the same direction as the evolutionary force of the chakra energies, let's look at the seven major chakras in more detail. The material presented here is based on my own research and has been found to apply to all my patients and to all workshop participants. It is offered as a starting point for your own experience and awareness.

The seven major chakras are located near specific organs in the physical body, more particularly the endocrine glands. They are linked by a central channel, known in Sanskrit as the *sushumna* (Fig. 17). The central channel is concurrent with the spine so that the seven main chakras appear to be embedded by their 'stems' very close to major nerve plexuses and certain endocrine glands.

The Base or Root Chakra

Located at the base of the spine. This centre is our link with nature and planet Earth. It deals with all issues of a physical nature – the body, the senses and sensuality, a person's sex, survival, aggression and self-defence.

At a physical level it is linked to the endocrine system through the adrenal glands. Its energies also affect the lower parts of the pelvis, the hips, legs and feet.

The chakra vibrates to the colour red, when in a state of balance. Like all chakra colours, it is seen with inner vision and is not identical with the colours of the physical spectrum. When seeking to obtain balance in any centre, the colours should be vibrant and without any area of shadow or darkness.

The Sacral Chakra

Opposite the sacral bones in the spine, between the navel and the base chakra. This chakra deals with all issues of creativity and sexuality (how we express ourselves sexually). It is the seat of joy and the place where the 'inner' child is originally located.

At the physical level, it is linked to the testes in the male and the ovaries in the female. Its energies also affect the uro-genital organs, the womb, the kidneys, the lower digestive organs and the lower back.

When in a state of balance, the sacral chakra vibrates to the colour orange.

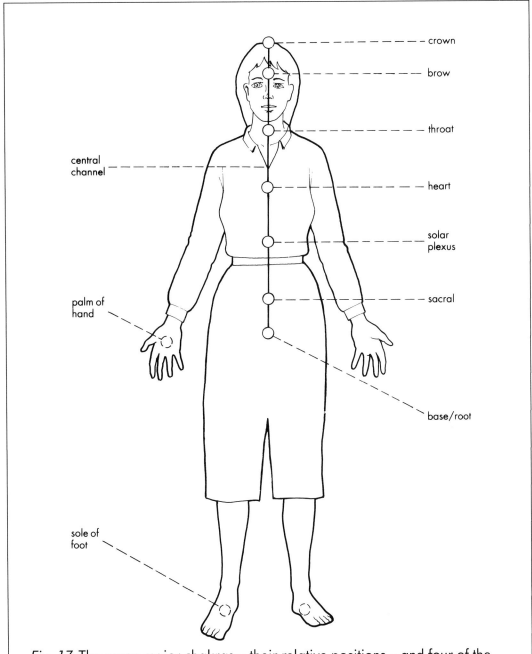

Fig. 17 The seven major chakras – their relative positions – and four of the minor chakras related to healing.

The Solar Plexus Chakra

Opposite the solar plexus, where we feel 'butterflies in the stomach'. Here the mind and personal will find expression. The 'lower' emotions based on fear – anxiety, insecurity, jealousy, anger, are generated here also, creating the important link between the mind and the emotions. What we think, whether positive or negative, has a great effect on our feelings and emotions. It is in the solar plexus chakra that negative energies related to thoughts and feelings are processed.

This is the place of the 'wounded child', though this child may also be found in the base or sacral chakras, according to the level of trauma which has prevented its emotional maturity.

At a physical level, the solar plexus chakra is linked to the Islets of Langerhans in the pancreas. Its energies also affect the solar and splenic nerve plexuses, the digestive system, the pancreas, liver, gall bladder, diaphragm (and so breathing), and middle back.

When in a state of balance, the solar plexus chakra vibrates to the colour yellow. This is a bright golden yellow.

The Heart Chakra

In the *centre* of the chest. This is the place of the soul, our inner guidance, and the seat of the 'higher' emotions based on unconditional love, such as empathy, compassion, true love, friendship, sister and brotherhood. At this level, feeling remains unconditioned by mind. The heart chakra deals with all issues concerned with love and affection, from the time of conception.

At a physical level, it is linked to the thymus gland. Its energies also affect the cardiac and pulmonary nerve plexuses, the heart, lungs, bronchial tubes, chest, upper back and arms.

When in a state of balance, the heart chakra vibrates to the colour green.

The Throat Chakra

Deals with all forms of communication and expression, whether through language, art, dance, music, and so on. This chakra also deals with the issue of truth and the true expression of the soul.

At a physical level, it is linked to the thyroid and parathyroid glands. Its energies also affect the pharyngeal nerve plexus, the organs of the throat, the neck, nose, mouth, teeth and ears. It is the chakra of the ears, nose and throat.

When in a state of balance, the throat chakra vibrates to the colour sky blue.

The Brow Chakra

In the middle of the forehead (inside the skull). The brow chakra is the place of intuition and soul knowledge. It oversees the activities of the chakras below it. It balances the power of mind and mental reasoning. It deals with the issues of developing and trusting intuition in our life, allowing soul knowledge through and developing and using high sense perception as a life skill.

At a physical level, it is linked to the hypothalamus and pituitary gland. Its energies also affect the nerves of the head, the brain, eyes and face.

When in a state of balance, the brow chakra vibrates to the colour indigo or royal blue.

The Crown Chakra

On the top of the head. This is the input centre for spiritual energies. It provides a direct link with the Source and deals with all issues of spirituality.

At a physical level, it is linked to the pineal gland (the light detector). Its energies also affect the brain and the rest of the body.

When in a state of balance, the crown chakra vibrates to the colour violet.

SENSING THE CHAKRAS

Now you can use the sensitivity you are developing to become aware of the chakras. Since the main system has a central place in all healing, it is essential for you to be able to locate where the seven major chakras are. Healthy chakras project energy so you should be able to sense this with your hand. If they need energizing, you may feel a response as energy *leaves* your palm in the direction of the chakra. Experiment with each palm to find out which is the most sensitive. This is the palm you will probably want to use in any sensing exercise. The exercises should be carried out with a partner.

EXERCISE 20: Sensing the Chakras to Locate Them

○ Your partner should sit comfortably in a chair with feet flat on the floor and hands on the thighs, with the elbows relaxed.

○ Stand at one side and hold your right hand about a forearm's width away from the front of your partner's body, with your palm opposite the base of the spine.

○ Bring your palm in towards your partner's body until you become aware of the sensation of energy flow in the region of the base chakra. You should still be a few inches away from the body and definitely not touching it. Do not worry if you cannot locate the chakra the first time, it will come with practice. Ask your partner if *your* energies can be sensed in the region of the base chakra. How does it feel?

○ Now gently move your hand up from this position until it is in line with the sacral area (opposite the sacral bones), just below the navel. See if you can locate the energy of the sacral chakra. Note any difference in sensation between one chakra and another.

○ Again, slowly and gently move your hand up until your palm is opposite your partner's solar plexus chakra, just above the navel. What do you sense this time?

○ Have a rest at this point and discuss with your partner what you both perceived. Your partner should remain seated in the same position, ready to continue the exercise when you are both focused again.

○ Hold your palm a few inches away from the centre of your partner's chest to sense the heart chakra. (This is not the same place as the physical heart.)

○ Gently move again to the throat, the brow and finally to a few inches above the crown chakra (Fig. 18).

○ Take time now to discuss your findings together before you change over roles, so that you may both fully share the complete experience of gently working with each other's etheric energy system.

Which directions do the chakras face, or do they face in all directions? The next exercise will help you find out the answer.

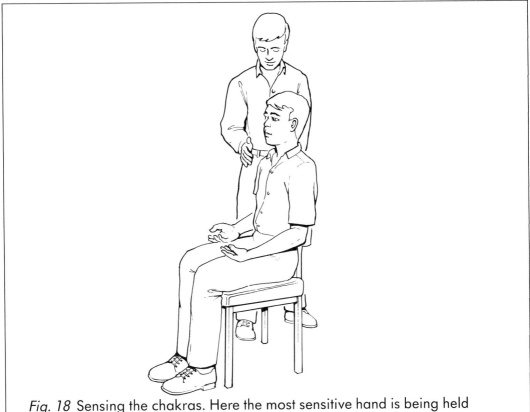

Fig. 18 Sensing the chakras. Here the most sensitive hand is being held opposite the throat chakra.

EXERCISE 21: Sensing the Chakras from Behind the Body

○ Have your partner sit sideways so that the back is free.

○ This time hold your palm at the back of your partner's body. Start opposite the base chakra and see if you can sense energy projecting in this direction. As before, move from chakra to chakra slowly and gently (a hasty movement at this level of concentration would sweep energy from one chakra to another, which is not the purpose of the exercise). After you have reached the crown chakra, discuss your findings together.

○ Make notes on any visual or other impressions which either of you may experience.

○ Repeat the exercise with your partner sitting in the normal way. Make a note of your discoveries.

YOUR INNER RAINBOW

As the energies of the etheric system move through the chakras they encompass the visible spectrum of seven colours. It should be remembered that the colours occur at an etheric level and tend to be very much more vibrant than the colours you see with normal vision. This movement of energy also symbolizes our own journey through the experiences of each chakra, each level of consciousness. As you deal with the issues which you encounter in the centres you are truly on a journey to the light through the human rainbow.

In the next exercise you will take a look at your inner rainbow. The actual colours you see, their quality and quantity will have much to tell you about the balance within your energy system and how this may relate to your current state of health. You can do this exercise alone.

EXERCISE 22: Sensing Colour in the Chakras

○ Sit or lie down comfortably. Allow yourself to relax and breathe slowly and normally.

○ Let your mind focus on the base chakra. Once it is there, allow yourself to 'see' what is on your internal 'screen'.

Do not expect it to be the colour red, it could be many other colours. It could be dark or cloudy or quite pale. It could be blotchy or uneven round the edge of your screen. Make a note of what you really sense or see with your inner vision.

○ Clear the screen and move your mind up to the sacral chakra. Make a note of what you sense or see there.

○ Clear the screen again and move from chakra to chakra until you reach the crown.

○ You now have a picture of what is actually going on in all your energy centres. When you bear in mind the colours to be found in each balanced chakra and the order in which they appear, any discrepancy is telling you something about the state of your system. This in turn, is saying something about you.

○ Decide what the different colours in your chakras mean. If, for example, there is orange in the solar plexus chakra, has your creativity or sexuality become an emotional issue? Green in the throat centre could mean that a love issue needs to be expressed, and so on. As you build up your findings you will begin to see that the colours have important messages for you, the healer.

○ How did this scan relate to what is going on in your life right now, the way you are feeling, your state of mind and health, etc.? Now try the exercise with a partner.

EXERCISE 23: Sensing Colour in the Chakras, with a Partner

This exercise involves working with a partner in a similar way.

○ Have your partner sit comfortably. This time your partner will tell you what s/he is experiencing as the focus moves from chakra to chakra.

○ To help your partner focus, hold your most sensitive palm a few inches away from the relevant chakra, starting at the base. You can hold your other palm near the back of the neck (opposite the throat chakra) to aid your partner's ability to express and communicate the impressions s/he receives (Fig. 19).

○ Move gently and slowly up through the system, making a note of what your partner senses each time. Discuss your findings together.

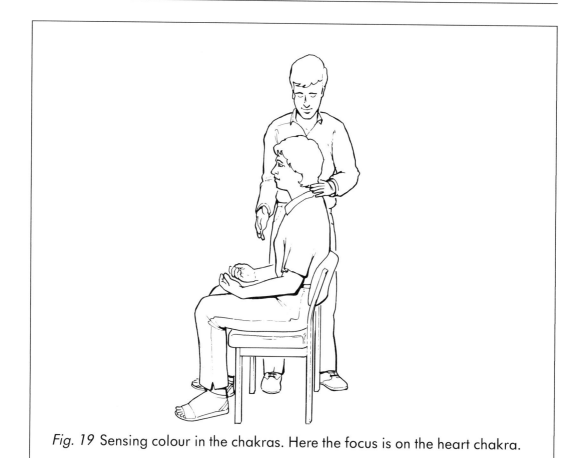

Fig. 19 Sensing colour in the chakras. Here the focus is on the heart chakra.

Working with a partner in this way shows you how you can use this as a healer to look at the balance of colours in your patient's energy system. It also demonstrates quite powerfully how you, as the healer, can help your patients to get in touch with their own inner messages.

You are on your way through the colours of the chakras. You may spend more time with one colour than another, because you need to. And at the end of this wonderful rainbow is the light that is you.

5

The Energies of
The Chakras

Jennifer was good at her job and she held a professional position with excellent career prospects. Her partner was just establishing himself in business, so her income provided the security they needed. Her first child was at nursery school. She also had a baby girl. After five months maternity leave she was able to return to her job by leaving the baby with a child minder.

Everything in Jennifer's life would have been going well if she could have got rid of her raging headaches and earache and the constant need to swallow. Her doctor had diagnosed blocked sinuses but had been unable to clear them. She tried homeopathy, which relieved the symptoms for a time, but the pain always returned, and with increasing intensity. Eventually she was having to take time off from her work.

Someone like Jennifer may come your way. If she decides to see a healer she will, of course, be wanting a cure for the pain in her head and ears, but at another level her energy system is calling for her to act in some way. Which chakra do you think is involved? The answer comes later. In the meantime, while you ponder on how you might help Jennifer, we will look at some of the other energies which your chakras process, over and above those discussed in Chapter 4.

THE FORCE OF EVOLUTION

As we make our way through life, the chakras call to us to confront the issues with which they deal. Each new experience gives us the opportunity to learn and to express, and the more we allow this to happen the clearer becomes the call from the crown chakra. This call is a spiritual force which draws the energies upwards – as if all our experiences are to culminate in unity with the Higher Self.

To help this process there is a store of spiritual energy lying dormant in the base chakra. It is a force of great potential which is generally awakened through spiritual practice and awareness. It has the power to link the levels of experience so that the soul's mission may be accomplished. This force is known by the Sanskrit word *kundalini*, another concept word which uses the image of serpent fire. The coiled serpent represents the potential nature of the force, and fire is its power to burn away stagnant energies trapped in the chakras. Though the whole image is benevolent, its great power requires appropriate respect.

When the kundalini is stimulated to rise in the central etheric channel, it assists in opening the chakras so that information from other levels can reach the mind. When the chakras have been developed in a systematic way, hand in hand with spiritual development, there is no problem in interpreting and using the new energies. This would not be the case, however, if the centres were opened through exercises alone (as they can be), for the personality would not be sufficiently evolved to be able to deal with the inrush of unfamiliar psychological material. This effect cannot occur if the exercises in this book are followed carefully and correctly.

Once we *are* in balance and the pathway to the crown chakra is clear, the kundalini may rise as a rush of energy up the spine. Various sensations may occur, ranging from light-headedness to a state of at-oneness or bliss.

Apart from its role as a vessel for the evolutionary force of kundalini, the other important task of the base chakra is to absorb and process energies from the planet which are also entering the system through the minor chakras of the feet.

Through the base chakra we are able to contact planetary wisdom and knowledge and the great teachings of nature. The chakras of the feet, in conjunction with the base chakra, allow us to earth or ground circuits which are set up during healing, meditation and other spiritual practices. When such activities have been completed and you wish to return to daily routine, a simple mental 'reconnection', such as becoming aware of the feet and toes, makes sure you do not continue with your 'head in the air'.

Planetary energies are relatively coarse compared with other energies within us, and they are drawn upwards to be further refined at each chakra.

THE FORCES OF VITALITY

Vitality energy from the cosmos enters the sacral chakra and mixes with the planetary energy. Vitality energy is essential to life and its particular function in the sacral chakra is to energize the forces of our sexuality and creativity. It also gives extra impetus to the child aspect of the Higher Self, to bring lightness of heart, fun and joy into our life. All energies being processed here are then drawn up to the solar plexus chakra for further refinement.

Here, the energies meet with the second and finer vitality energy. This has great energizing properties which act on the physical body and also give power to the feelings and force to the mind, to project thought energy. The energies of the lower three chakras are processed here before moving upward to the heart chakra.

THE FORCE OF BALANCE

The heart chakra is the balancing centre of the seven main chakras, for it also processes spiritual energies moving downwards from the three chakras above it. Energy moving upwards needs to be refined and processed in the heart centre before moving on its way to the crown chakra. Only then can it be effectively used by the higher centres. Similarly, energy moving down through the system needs to be processed by the heart chakra so that it can be used effectively by the lower centres.

Significantly, the heart chakra vibrates to the colour green, the colour of balance. We are aware that all the issues of the heart centre, mentioned earlier, are critical to human evolution at the present time. We know that our problems can only be solved by the energies of the heart chakra and the wisdom that they represent. The human race has tried to solve issues through the solar plexus, under the limited guidance of the mind. This has meant drawing on the powers of will, force and violence, which are all based on fear and the sense of separation. These methods have failed over and over again. To progress we have to move up to the heart chakra and open up to the power of love, understanding and compassion to solve our problems.

The heart centre has the answer because it is the place of the soul. Here we can access the wisdom of the Higher Self. If the answer was in our minds we would have discovered it already, but first we have to learn about the limitations of the mind. The mind is conditioned and cannot apply knowledge with love, only the heart can do this.

How or whether we love each other, care for others, whether we share or have a lifestyle based on fear rather than love and trust – such issues are knocking at all our doors. These are some of the issues being brought to healers today. So often a particular problem has its roots in whether people love themselves, are able to give love, or receive love. In all areas of our lives we find ourselves confronted by the choice to live by fear or by love. Whatever we choose will have to find expression, and this is through the throat chakra.

THE FORCE OF SELF-EXPRESSION

The force of the throat chakra is to encourage us to communicate and express all the energies that are moving up from the chakras below it as well as the spiritual energies moving down from the brow and crown centres. The throat centre offers us the challenge to be true to ourselves and express who and what we truly are. When we do not do this or when energy is prevented from flowing freely in this centre, an energy block will develop.

Jennifer wanted a cure for her headaches, earache, blocked sinuses and blocked nose and, during the initial part of the healing session, hinted that she suspected a deep-seated cause which she could not identify. The chakra scan revealed that there was no energy leaving her throat centre at all – there was a block in it.

She said she had no problem in expressing or communicating at work, she was good at it. Was there a problem at home then? As she registered the question in her mind her throat chakra began to absorb healing energy from my hand, signalling that the home was the seat of the block.

As the healing continued she was able to express how she felt torn between going to work, continuing her career, and being with the children. As she talked, so the throat chakra took in more and more energy.

After the first session, Jennifer's symptoms began to subside. The healing showed her that her personality wanted her to carry on working, but her inner

Self wanted her to be with her children. As part of the healing, she was able to express what she really wanted and come to a decision.

With her husband she worked out a satisfactory compromise and she now works part-time. Her terrible head pains have subsided and the sinus condition has almost cleared. Jennifer realized that her sinus issue was her body's way of telling her when she was not expressing herself (when she was blocking her throat chakra).

THE FORCE OF INTUITION

How did you get on with your interpretation of Jennifer's condition? Did you let your intuition guide you or did you try to puzzle it out? The intuitive force is soul knowledge, which is processed by the brow chakra. The brow chakra impresses us with intuitive information which is outside of the mind's storehouse of knowledge. This is why intuitive information so often seems strange, unfamiliar, even unbelievable.

Sometimes we act on our 'hunches', but all too often the mind's analysis gets in the way. By allowing intuition to play a more positive role in life, this problem is gradually overcome.

As healers develop, their chakras become more open. In the case of the brow chakra this means that, as high sense perception increases, ways of sensing finer vibrations become enhanced. Clairvoyance, for example, is a typical by-product of brow chakra development. This is why the chakra has been known historically and in many cultures as the 'third eye'.

THE FORCE OF THE SOUL

As we respond to the call of the soul to acknowledge our mission, our reason for being here, the crown chakra opens up to absorb more spiritual energy. This will be used to upgrade the entire energy system and it is what prompts the potential force of kundalini in the base chakra to rise and assist in the process.

ENERGY BLOCKS AND THEIR EFFECTS

Each chakra is a repository of wisdom related to its many functions. Getting in touch with the wisdom of the centres presents new possibilities for self-healing and for bringing others to balance and harmony. However, our ability to work with these possibilities can be hampered by barriers we may encounter at many levels. These often take the form of energy blocks.

An energy block in a chakra may have far reaching effects. On the subtle levels it can have a detrimental effect on the areas and issues with which the chakra deals. A person may experience problems in releasing or getting in touch with their creativity, for example, because of a block in the sacral chakra, the solar plexus, heart, or all three.

On a physical level it may affect areas of the physical body which it influences through its connection, via the relevant endocrine glands, with the surrounding organs and tissues.

Stan, who was mentioned in Chapter 4, had a block in the solar plexus chakra which acted on his pancreas to prevent him from properly metabolizing insulin. In Jennifer's case, her blocked throat chakra affected the sinuses, ears, nose and throat.

Energy blocks are our own responsibility because they are self-induced. Part of the healer's task is to show patients how they have blocked their own system so that they can understand how their condition has occurred. Later in the book we shall be looking again at how healing can help people release energy blocks.

The following exercise puts the chakras in a state of balance, though the effect is temporary. It should not be used before any work to *discover* where energy blocks are located. Practise the exercise with a partner.

EXERCISE 24: Balancing the Chakras

○ Have your partner sit comfortably, relax and breathe normally. You are going to bring pure white light down through your partner's crown chakra and gently on through the rest of the other major chakras to balance the system.

○ Stand at one side of your partner and raise your hands above his or her head with the palms facing inward, about a shoulder's width apart. Ask for the pure light of spiritual energy to be directed down to your partner (Fig. 20).

○ Slowly bring your hands in until they are an inch or two from your partner's head, but not touching the head. Keep your hands at this distance from the body throughout the exercise. You may be able to sense the light when it arrives as a tingling in the palms. Ask your partner if s/he can sense the energy as it is moved gently down to the crown chakra.

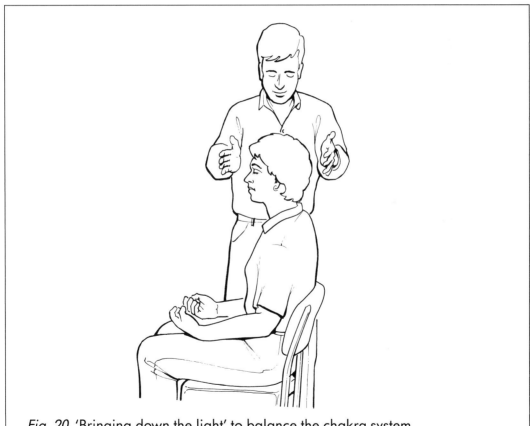

Fig. 20 'Bringing down the light' to balance the chakra system.

○ Gently and slowly move your hands together down towards the brow chakra. Ask your partner if there are any sensations as the light passes through. There may be a feeling of resistance. This probably indicates an energy block. If so, ask your partner to 'let go' to allow the light through. Do not rush this movement.

○ Move your hands together down either side of your partner's body, as you visualize the white light passing through each chakra in turn.

○ Check each time that there is no resistance. If there is, again, ask your partner to 'let go' in that area and allow the light through.

○ Finally, draw the light out at the base chakra. The energy system is now in a state of balance.

This exercise should not be carried out if you wish to look into the state of a patient's balance (as in *Sensing Colour in the Chakras*, Exercise 22), but it is a useful exercise to do afterwards.

RELEASING THE BLOCK

If we think of the chakra system in terms of our own progress, we can see that any block in the system will announce itself when we are working on our personal development or on developing healing potential. Healers, for example, need a heart chakra where the energy of unconditional love is able to flow freely. If they have experienced emotional trauma which has created a block in the solar plexus, thus impeding the flow to the heart chakra, the block will need to be healed.

Wherever an energy block is located it can have a range of effects. A block *between* chakras can prevent the free flow of energy in the subtle channels which can inhibit the growth of the personality. For example, a block between the base and sacral chakras may slow down sexual maturity and the full expression of physicality.

Once we understand this aspect of the chakra system, we can begin to work on our own energy blocks and also take steps to prevent them. The following exercise, which can be performed daily, helps to clear the chakras and to balance them. It also gives you clues to those which are being adversely affected in some way or to issues which need addressing.

EXERCISE 25: Balancing Your Own Chakra System

○ First visualize a column of pure white light above your head.

○ As you breathe in, draw this light down until it 'hovers' above your crown chakra.

○ On the next in-breath, allow the light to pass through the crown chakra and straight down the central channel, through each chakra in turn. Do this slowly and gently, co-ordinating it with your breathing.

○ Pause when you feel any resistance and wait until you are able to proceed. You can practise 'letting go' or getting in touch with the energy of the resistance. This means focusing on the area of resistance.

○ Relax and sense if anything comes up on your internal screen. This may give a clue to what the energy block is about. The clue will tell you what or who you need to let go of.

The next exercise will refresh you. It clears away other vibrations in the system which are not compatible with your own and initiates a process of energy regulation within the system which brings about balance. You are 'fine tuning' your chakras through the use of colour breathing. The exercise co-ordinates the breath with colour visualization to cleanse and adjust the whole energy system.

EXERCISE 26: Regulating the Chakras

○ Sit or lie comfortably. Relax and breathe gently and normally.

○ Allow your mind to drop slowly to the base centre. Look at your internal 'screen'. Try to see the colour red as a light with a slight tinge of bright pink in it.

○ Whatever you see that is different to this is telling you what is going on at this level. For example, any darkness will indicate a build up of energy which needs to be processed, while a pale shade indicates a lack of energy in this chakra.

○ Now co-ordinate your breathing with colour. On the in-breath, breathe in the red light until the base chakra is vibrating to a bright, clear colour. Note any difficulties you have in bringing in the vibrant colour and any variations which were in the centre before you worked to change it.

○ Clear your screen and move the mind up to the sacral chakra. Visualize a bright orange light. Use the in-breath to breathe in orange until your centre glows with this colour. Again, note any difficulties in achieving the colour.

○ Clear the screen again and move the mind up to the solar plexus chakra. Breathe in a golden yellow light.

○ Move to the heart centre in the same way as before and breathe in a fresh green light.

○ Move to the throat centre and breathe in a clear sky blue (note any clouds!).

○ Move to the brow chakra and breathe in an indigo light (this colour should be vivid and not dark).

○ Move to the crown and breathe in a violet light.

○ Now look at what you have recorded. What were the particular areas of difficulty? The exercise can be repeated until the clarity of the colours improves. Its effect on the energies is to regulate them by acting on their actual flow and speed of vibration.

The next exercise equips you to help your patients regulate their energy systems in the same way. The procedure is the same as in the previous exercise but done with a partner.

EXERCISE 27: Regulating the Chakras with a Partner

○ Your partner should sit comfortably and take two full breaths while relaxing the body.

○ Hold your most sensitive palm near your partner's base chakra to help process the energy. Do not touch your partner's body with the hand during this exercise.

○ As in the previous exercise, your partner breathes in red light while focusing on the base chakra.

○ When as much of this colour as possible has been breathed into the chakra, move on to the next chakra. Continue the exercise, moving slowly and gently up the system.

○ Ask if there are any difficulties in achieving the relevant colours. Note any changes in the energies you may have sensed in the palms as (a) your partner focused on the chakra and (b) the energy was being processed.

NOTE: Colour breathing is best done during the hours of daylight. This is because the system is 'at rest' during the night, when colour breathing would stimulate it to be active.

CLOSING DOWN THE CHAKRAS

The chakras allow the intake of energies vital to life, so they are never totally closed. Their capacity is usually increased (they are opened) through stimulation such as spiritual disciplines, meditation, healing, prayer and any form of colour breathing such as in the above exercise. This is useful, for it increases chakra activity and capacity for absorption of energies. Once these activities have ceased, however, it is essential to 'close down' the system to reduce the capacity for energy absorption and to limit chakra activity to normal levels again. This does not mean that the chakras should ever be closed completely, for this would be detrimental to health.

I was given a dramatic illustration of this by a patient who had come for healing with a series of nervous complaints. He had symptoms of chronic energy loss, weight loss and suffered severe headaches from time to time. He was 35 but looked 20 years older. He had no idea what the problem was and his medical specialist had done his best to address each symptom with little result.

The first healing session revealed blocks in five chakras and underfunctioning in two others. I was puzzled and asked him what had been going on.

'That's just it, I don't know. I used to practise yoga on a regular basis, but I've stopped that now. I still remember to close down every day before going to work though.'

I asked him how he 'closed down' and his reasons for doing so.

'I imagine my centres closing tight shut. This protects me during the day so that I won't lose any vital energy.'

Here was the clue to my patient's very poor condition. He had learned about closing down the chakras from a friend, and had consciously set about closing each chakra as firmly as possible to 'protect himself'. This had been going on for over a year, reducing his intake of vital energies quite drastically. The result was a gradual deterioration in health and wellbeing.

I explained to him the effect of completely closing his chakras for so long and suggested exercises to 'open' them, and a programme of colour breathing to raise their energy levels. Within a week he was feeling better and within two months had regained his former good health.

The following exercise is a safe way to close down (rather than shut up) the system and should be used after any sessions of exercises with the book from now on, if you are intending to return to everyday tasks. This is part of your responsibility to yourself and towards the energies with which you are dealing. If you take up healing as a profession, responsible attitudes are essential at all times.

EXERCISE 28: Closing Down

For the purpose of this exercise, visualize your chakras as somewhat like flowers with petals that close up at night, but not tightly. After completing your work or exercises, see the 'flowers' of each chakra gently closing up a little. The exercise can be down either standing or sitting.

○ Start at the crown chakra and close it down a little.

○ Move on to the brow chakra.

○ Slowly move down the system until you reach the base chakra.

With practice this exercise is done in a moment or two.

Another way to close down the system is to say a prayer of thanks either mentally or aloud. Remember that if you do another exercise, some healing, or even read a spiritually orientated book, your chakras could be opened again, and you will need to repeat the closing down exercise.

DISPERSING INCOMPATIBLE ENERGIES

The Rainbow Breath is a cleansing breath which clears the aura, dispersing incompatible energies, and has a directly beneficial effect on the subtle bodies. It is an excellent exercise to do after spiritual work or at the end of the day.

EXERCISE 29: The Rainbow Breath

○ Stand with your feet a shoulder-width apart with your arms held loosely at your sides.

○ Do some *Full Breath Breathing* three times. Let your shoulders drop and

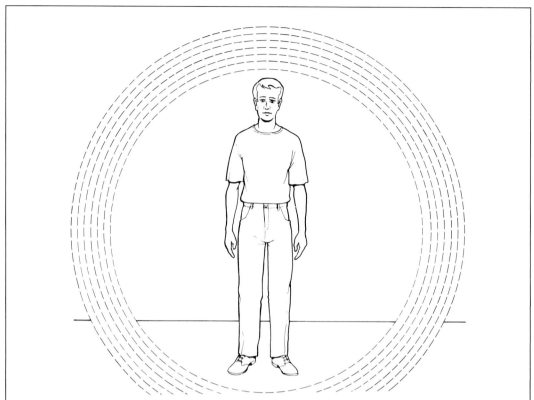

Fig. 21 The Rainbow Breath – surrounding yourself with seven spheres of light to clear and balance the aura.

relax your body. On the out-breath let go of any worries and anxieties. Send the message to your body that this is a treat for the whole system.

○ Now visualize that you can enclose yourself with seven spheres of coloured light in the following way. Breathe in slowly and deeply. As you do so, see red light rising from behind your heels, moving up your legs and up to the top of your head.

○ On the out-breath see the red light moving down over the front of your body until it is under your feet. You are now enclosed in a sphere of red light.

○ Breathe up orange light and surround your red sphere with it in the same way, making sure that it totally encloses the red sphere and creates an orange sphere outside it.

○ Breathe up yellow light and surround the orange sphere.

○ Breathe up green and surround the yellow sphere.

○ Breathe up blue and surround the green sphere.

○ Breathe up indigo and surround the blue sphere.

○ Breathe up violet and surround the indigo sphere. You are now totally enclosed in a wonderful rainbow of light (Fig. 21). Without moving, go straight on with the next exercise.

You can follow up the last exercise with the *Sphere of Protection*. This is an outer layer of golden light with which you surround your aura and, if used in conjunction with the *Rainbow Breath*, it is the final outermost sphere.

EXERCISE 30: The Sphere of Protection

○ On the in-breath, breathe up a bright golden light and surround yourself with a sphere of gold on the out-breath. This is an energy of strength and protection. It allows positive vibrations into your aura, but prevents negative ones from entering (Fig. 22).

Use this exercise at the end of the day or at any time when you feel the need for protection. It is a good exercise to do at the end of a workshop on personal development or a meditation session when you are going to return to everyday life.

The *Sphere of Protection* can be used on its own whenever you feel the need to protect yourself or use it with the exercises of *Closing Down* and the *Rainbow Breath* to form a routine for the end of your day. With practice they can be done within seconds.

The *Rainbow Breath* does not involve your breathing *in* colour so it is quite safe to do during the hours of darkness.

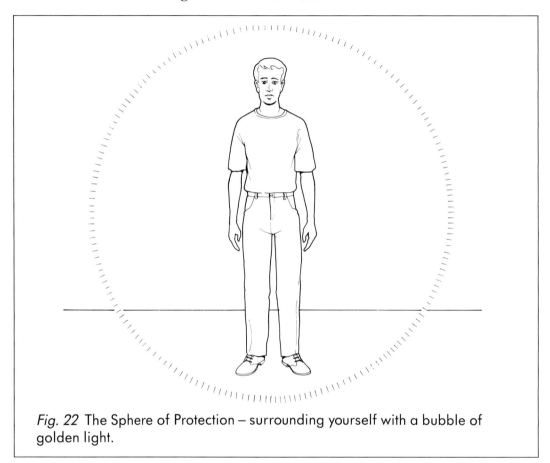

Fig. 22 The Sphere of Protection – surrounding yourself with a bubble of golden light.

Having worked with the energies and built up some basic knowledge of the energy pattern that goes to make *you,* you are ready to look at how to work with the energies to heal your life and bring about positive change.

6

The Wisdom of The Body and Causes of Ill Health

*J*oan had a history of back trouble. Osteopathy helped her a great deal, but the pain in her lower back would sooner or later return. During her first healing session, Joan was asked about the stresses in her life. She said she had a very interesting and well-paid job, but her boss was very demanding and domineering. He had a knack of knowing how to put her down whenever she did her work particularly well.

On reflection she could remember that her back would go into spasm within a day or two after one of her boss's verbal put-downs. The healer encouraged her to get in touch with her lower back to see if it could tell her more about the problem. As she relaxed, the healer directed healing to her lower back.

Into Joan's mind came scene after scene of humiliation. Her anger and her distress were unexpressed and stored in the lower back. She had found no way of releasing the energies so they reacted on one of the weakest parts of her body, her lower back. In this way, her body had been able to prevent her from going to work and incurring more of the same treatment. It was trying to draw her attention to a problem which needed to be solved. This gave Joan a fresh perspective on the pain she had been going through.

She was later encouraged to get in touch with why she could not assert her right to be and why she allowed her boss to repeatedly humiliate her. Healing helped her to start loving and valuing herself. Her new attitude meant that her boss was also forced to confront his own inadequate behaviour.

SYMPTOMS AS SIGNALS

The function of disease is to draw our attention to any state of imbalance. It is our body's signal that we need to address the situation. If we insist on masking the symptoms which are the body's signals, it will try again to sound the alarm in another way. It does this because it is part of us, it is our friend and can be trusted. Its ultimate message may be that we are cut off from the Self.

The difference between allopathic medicine and spiritual healing reflects the way these disciplines each approach, perceive and treat a person's body. Traditional medicine works with the symptoms of a condition and seeks to alleviate them.

Healing looks at the whole person, seeing them as spirit, mind, emotions and body, in that order, and works with the cause and meaning of their ill health as well as the condition itself. It also proceeds from a position of confidence that each person holds the key to his or her own healing. Part of the healer's role, then, is to help people get in touch with the body's wisdom, to activate their own healing potential. For many, this will be a radical change to the way they usually regard themselves.

Sometimes we might reject certain friends only to rebuild the friendship at a later date. Perhaps you need to do this with your body. The body is your ally. It is never your enemy. The following exercises will help you get to know your friend a little better and to realize that it is a friend to be respected and trusted. Aches and pains are often the physical sign of energy imbalance at some level. By getting in touch with the body's signals you can gain insight which will help you restore balance.

EXERCISE 31: Working with Aches and Pains

○ Sit or lie comfortably. Breathe slowly and relax the body.

○ Starting with your feet, scan your body for places where you feel discomfort of any kind.

○ When you locate such a place, let your attention relax into it; take your time. Allow yourself to fully feel the discomfort while remaining as relaxed as possible.

○ Tell yourself that you wish to understand the cause of the discomfort and to penetrate beyond what may seem obvious. You are talking to the cells of this area of your body. Wait patiently for their reply. Make a note of any impressions you receive, however strange they may seem.

○ Move on to the next place of discomfort and proceed in the same way.

○ When you have scanned the whole body, send it a message of thanks.

○ Finally put all your impressions and information together. You may see a pattern emerging or you may gain insight into the present state of your body which will guide you in providing the best treatment.

   Perhaps your body indicated that the problem actually has its origin at another level. Perhaps you have been upset or under stress and the mental or emotional aspects of your being are out of alignment. This will be your first consideration when beginning self-healing.

Like Joan, our response to life's challenges is not always as positive as we would like and there are many reasons for this. The following exercise can be used whenever you are confronted with a problem and your difficulty in coping with it. The body is a repository of wisdom. Through the network of consciousness it has access to the other levels of your being from which you may have cut yourself off. By linking with the body consciousness, you can tap into this valuable source of inner guidance.

EXERCISE 32: Using Body Wisdom in Problem Solving

○ Sit or lie comfortably. Breathe slowly and gently as you relax your body.

○ Note where you feel tension in your body. Remain aware of these areas as you let go and release the tension from them.

○ Ask your body to help you in coping with your particular problem. Tell it whether your need is for insight or some sort of solution.

○ Now let the problem drift from your mind into your body. Let it move anywhere in the body until it comes to rest.

○ Relax your attention into this place in your body where your problem's energies are gathered. Wait patiently for the still small voice within to talk to you. The response may not be verbal. Be prepared for the unexpected and accept your body's response with good grace.

○ Thank your body and make a note of your answer.

○ See the problem once more gathered up as a 'ball' of energy. Breathe in peace. Release the energies of the problem and breathe them out.

○ Repeat the breathing pattern until you feel the problem is fully cleared from your body.

COMING TO TERMS WITH STRESS

A certain amount of stress keeps us in touch with life. Our evolution as human beings gives us an inbuilt ability to cope with a level of stress, so that it can be life-enhancing. The body is very well equipped to do this, and the wisdom of the body will try to alert us to situations which may threaten to overpower its ability to cope.

Sometimes we ignore the body's early warning signals, such as minor aches and pains, and wait until stress has induced disease before we decide to act and bring about necessary changes.

Rapid changes in the modern environment and the way we live and work have created new stress factors which no longer help us to interact with life situations in a productive way. They are in fact life-threatening. What we perceive as stress overload can seriously affect the balance of our energies and bring about ill health. So we need to look carefully at the stresses in our lives and decide which ones we can eliminate or change, and how to devise positive coping strategies for those we cannot change.

We have to come to terms with stress, for our response to it and how we are able to change will determine the amount of stress we experience. Stress means different things to different people and we differ in our inborn capacities to cope. When we have to face events in our lives which are important or painful to us, we have to make a great effort to adjust. The amount of effort we need to put in will have a bearing on the amount of stress we experience.

For example, a person who understands the soul's journey will be better able to let go of a loved one when they pass over, in spite of suffering the stress of loss and the pain of grieving. But the person who sees death as final and cannot easily let go will probably suffer even more stress and prolong the grieving process because of how death affects them. In the latter case, the state of imbalance which persists for a longer time, may adversely influence physical health.

Change is a key element in our growth and development, for only through change can we learn. But fear of change can prevent us from adapting to it successfully. This failure to respond in a positive way, to create a positive coping strategy, is at the root of many forms of stress.

In our response to change we can identify two main types of stress effects. In the first, we feel under stress, but the surge of energy and enthusiasm, produced by the added adrenalin in the system, helps us to get going and get things done. When we harness this response to a definite aim, stress is constructive.

On another occasion, the demands on us may exceed our capacity to adjust or harness the response. Then the stress becomes destructive and is often experienced as pain on a physical, mental, or emotional level, or on a combination of levels.

WHAT IS STRESS?

On the physical level, stress comes from outside us in the form of pollution, poor housing, poor nutrition, other environmental factors or a stress-filled lifestyle. The emotional pressures of partners, friends, family, our love life, environmental factors affecting us at this level, can add to the physical stresses we are trying to cope with. The mind, in trying to deal with the stresses mentioned above, may also be put under intolerable pressures.

Many such stresses quickly become internalized so that they, in turn, develop as stresses within. Because of the energy imbalances this induces, we may become ill in body, mind or spirit.

We can increase stress levels and imbalance from within by the way we behave. When our behaviour produces negative or destructive effects on us, this is a self-abuse of body, emotions or mind.

We can abuse our bodies through diet, smoking, use of drugs, lack of exercise, and so on. The emotions can be abused by the continued exercise of negative emotions or by using our emotions in destructive ways. Fears and phobias, anxiety and worry, all create stress and imbalance on the emotional level and in the astral and etheric bodies.

Most fear and anxiety originates at a mental level and is the result of negative thinking. Because the mind and lower emotions operate together through the solar plexus chakra, they create a powerful force of negativity which can have far-reaching and destructive effects on the etheric and physical bodies.

Negative thinking is an abuse of mind and this abuse accounts for most of the horror and distress we see in human life at this time. We have to remember that negative thoughts are attracted to each other. When enough force has been gathered, they act on the physical level to produce the negative effects we experience around us.

The abuse of mind and the abuse of our power centre, the solar plexus chakra, creates stresses and imbalances which will require great control to counteract. Such is the power and effect of the mind that we can literally think ourselves into illness. But, conversely, this power can be used to think ourselves *out* of illness and into good health.

IDENTIFYING PERSONAL STRESS

It is important for healers to be able to help people identify their stress and also to define it. Your body can help you do this. In the following exercise you will need to let your body speak to you, to help you make this discovery. Let your attitude be one of trust, respect and anticipation.

EXERCISE 33: Identifying Stress

○ Sit comfortably and close your eyes. Take a few deep breaths.

○ Recall a situation you found yourself in which you did not like and with which you did not cope very well.

○ Allow your body to remind you about how you felt and to show you how you responded. Try to recall the experience with a certain amount of detachment, so that you can make a note of your responses. Did you react physically, emotionally, mentally or a combination of these?

You could have felt pain in your body or in the mind. You may have felt agitated, under pressure, unable to cope, and so on. Note down as much as you can.

○ Finally, thank yourself for showing you the stressful situation.

○ Concentrate on your breathing again. Put one hand on the solar plexus chakra (just above the navel) and breathe slowly and deeply.

○ Breathe in love. Breathe out the situation. Keep breathing like this until you feel the condition is cleared from your body.

EXERCISE 34: Identifying Stress Effects

○ Go into a stressful situation, as in the previous exercise. Let your body talk to you again, but this time take the exercise a stage further.

○ Ask your body to show you the effects of what you have experienced in terms of what the energies are doing in your system.

○ Then ask it to show you the possible longer term results of these effects. This will give you insight into how your body will probably deal with the energies.

○ Proceed to let go of the situation as in the previous exercise.

THE FUNCTION OF STRESS

When we identify a situation as needing our immediate attention the body goes into a series of reactions which are designed to meet the need. At the extremes of stress we could be under attack or feel under severe pressure due to the messages which are being processed by the brain.

The hypothalamus stimulates the pituitary gland to release hormones which in turn activate the adrenal glands. As the level of adrenalin in the bloodstream goes up, heart rate increases and there is increased blood supply to the brain and muscles. Breathing rate increases and extra carbohydrates are released into the blood to provide extra energy. This and other reactions have prepared the body for 'fight or flight'. We are at a peak of arousal.

This level of arousal may be uncomfortable, as when we experience 'butterflies in the stomach', but it is very valuable when we need to go into action. A person about to give some sort of performance, for example, needs these body reactions to produce their best. Part of the art of performance is learning how to use the body's state of readiness and not to let fear or anxiety – which are sensed in the solar plexus – paralyse and de-activate us.

Sometimes we are ready to act but we cannot or are unable to do so. The person caught in a long traffic jam would like to drive out of the situation. Assessment of the problem gives the choice of a good coping strategy such as listening to the radio or studying passers-by, or a negative coping strategy such as seeing the situation as a stressful one, worrying about being late, a missed meeting, various negative repercussions at the other end of the journey. These worries and anxieties activate the hormone system to do something, but the 'victim' still cannot act. Stress increases due to this limitation and the negative coping strategy takes its toll.

DEALING WITH STRESS-RELATED IMBALANCES

When someone's lifestyle means that they are constantly wound up to act at peak performance only to have this frustrated in various ways, the body has to cope with trying to wind down the processes it has put into action. The stresses felt by the person have brought about further imbalances at the etheric level and also at the emotional and mental levels.

The toll on the body is perhaps easier to understand. The constantly increasing heartbeat, for example, with the bloodstream becoming overloaded with unused components, could lead to a knock-on effect on the heart, circulatory system and perhaps other organs and other systems.

At the etheric level, there is a build up of energy in the solar plexus chakra which could lead to energy blockage when repeated over and over again. Emotional and mental turmoil create further imbalances, which affect the pattern of thought and feeling as the energies filter down to the etheric level.

Via the chakras and meridians, these negative messages soon reach every cell in the body.

This is unproductive stress and its effects on us will be destructive both in the short and the long term. Therefore, we should have a healthy respect for the effects of our negative coping strategies and what unreleased stress can do to us. Symptoms are many and range from disorders in the digestive, circulatory, respiratory, endocrine, nervous and immune systems to symptoms such as nervous movements, habits, apathy and irritability. The build up of unreleased stress can also cause or exacerbate conditions such as asthma, skin disorders, depression, ME and cancer.

The way to avoid stress-related illness is to get to know yourself intimately and without fear so that you can create strategies which will work to your benefit. If you are working with others, you will need to find ways to help them understand and appreciate their own responses, so that together you can creative positive outcomes.

STRESS AND PERSONALITY

When looking at the way energy imbalance is brought about through stress, it is important to recognize that we all vary in our vulnerability and in our reaction to stress. There are factors in our personality and in our conditioning which play an important part in determining how we will respond. Hippocrates (born c. 460 B.C.) was one of the first great therapists to link personality type to health and wellbeing.

This link is the key to modern thinking about stress management and control. It suggests that our vulnerability to stress is to be found in the personality and the factors, both genetic and developmental, which have gone into its making.

This is the sum total of personality that researchers are working with when they investigate our responses to stress. The research of Friedman and Rosenman in the early 1960s, for example, highlighted two main patterns of behaviour which they describe as Type A and Type B personalities (see Further Reading).

Type A people show a high rate of coronary heart disease. They are often competitive, aggressive, ambitious, impatient and restless people. They converse rapidly, frequently interrupting, and find it difficult to listen to others. They are physically tense and ruled by the clock. Type A people see other

Type A's as a challenge. Hostility is not far from the surface. They cannot play without seeing the 'game' as a contest. If they have time to spare they feel guilty 'doing nothing'.

Type B people have a low rate of coronary heart disease. They are more relaxed, are laid back and are better listeners. They are not inclined to hurry or create deadlines. Type B people are free of Type A traits. They do not harbour hostility and can relax and have fun without needing to demonstrate some sort of achievement.

Are you one of these types or are you perhaps a mixture of the two? Whatever you are, the research suggests that you should look at the characteristics of the Type B personality and try to bring more elements of this type into your life and lifestyle.

You need to look at your job, the workplace, your lifestyle and the things you have to deal with, in terms of how stressful *you* find them. Some coping strategies may be inborn, but most can be learned. Negative coping strategies add to the problem. They range from alcohol and drugs to depression and compulsive habits. Denial of a situation is the worst form of coping strategy because this allows for no way forward.

There are many positive coping strategies. The best is to have some spiritual healing because this will address all levels of imbalance. Breathing exercises, relaxation, meditation and visualization, as described in this book, will all develop a basis for coping with stress in a positive way.

Look at the way you feel about yourself and try to judge yourself more favourably, if you have to pass judgement at all. You need to talk about your stress and communicate how you are feeling to a sympathetic ear. Finally, you may need to replan your life, make time for breaks, hobbies, having fun.

If you are already telling yourself this is a tall order, the chances are you are a Type A person! We are responsible for our own health and wellbeing so it is up to us to take the necessary steps to eradicate the harmful effects of stress in our lives.

By working with the wisdom of the body, as set out in the exercises throughout this book, you will be able to create a positive life plan which will be a blueprint for your own healing.

7

Change, The Mind and Emotions

*R*achel began to cough. She interrupted her first healing session to ask
for a glass of water. 'I wonder if I should come back another time?'
she spluttered.

My hand was opposite her solar plexus chakra to where I was directing
healing. I reassured her, realizing that it would have been a way for
Rachel to avoid continuing with the healing. I suggested she finish her
drink and see if she could complete the session.

'I always cough when I'm nervous,' she said. 'I cough when I'm with a
group of people. Then I can leave the room to get a drink, I can get away
from the situation.'

'That's interesting, because the cough draws their attention to you. So
it's a plea for attention as well as a way of escaping. Are you feeling
nervous right now?'

'No, I just feel uncomfortable. That's what starts me coughing.'

Rachel had sought healing to deal with an inexplicable nervousness
which was badly affecting her personal and professional life. The cause of
her nervousness appeared to be deeply embedded in her solar plexus
chakra. As soon as healing was directed there, she began to cough. She
was getting in touch with the root of the problem.

A recent change of job was the current focus for Rachel's nervousness.
She felt afraid in new social situations and was nervous about not being
able to cope. The healing helped her to identify that her nervousness was

in fact a fear of not being in control. Her cough was a signal about coping with change and losing control. She further identified that this was her response to all forms of change in her life.

Rachel's cough originated at the level of the mind and the emotions. Whenever her mind registered that any change was imminent it generated feelings of fear. These in turn triggered her cough. In subsequent healing sessions she was able to understand the childhood origin of her fear from which she was helped to grow away.

THE SURVIVAL PURPOSE OF FEAR

Nature shows us that life is change, that nothing stays the same. As we saw in Chapter 6, change is a fact of life, but it can often be the cause of stress. From the moment of birth, we need food, care and attention, and love. If, for any reason, we do not get enough of these vital nourishments, we know fear. So fear drives us to try to obtain what we need in order to survive.

But the survival purpose of fear soon begins to permeate all aspects of life as we become aware that, apparently, there is no endless source of anything. We are taught by fearful parents and carers to live by the fear of lack and loss. Like those who condition us, we align our lives with these fears, cutting ourselves off from the source of what we need. This is where our fear of change, and our resistance to change, originates, and this where much energy imbalance begins.

THE POWER OF MIND AND EMOTIONS

We all have to come to terms with change and it is the mind and the emotions that influence our ability to change. We saw how important the role of mind was in addressing causes of stress and in the way it could generate further stress. Because of its link with the emotions in the solar plexus chakra, the mind has a powerful influence on the way we express our feelings and on the emotions these may arouse.

The mind generates thoughts which may be positive or negative. We always have a choice in how we wish to think, though past conditioning, unless addressed, will influence our tendency to make positive or negative choices. For example, you look out of the window and see it raining. You look at the grey clouds and think: 'What miserable weather. I was going to go for a walk, but I can't now.' Or you may think: 'We need water. The plants need water to grow. I'm not going to let the rain spoil my day. I'll put on a mac and enjoy the feeling of the rain on my face.' While a more detached view might be to simply watch the rain, noting the changes in the sky, deciding whether or not to go for a walk, but feeling perfectly equanimous about it.

These three possible positions show how our thinking can affect mood and attitudes. But at all times we can choose how to think. We need to remember that like begets like and that positive attitudes beget positive feelings which beget positive actions. In this way the mind affects how we choose to behave.

For example, you are driving your car when someone carelessly swerves in front of you, causing you to brake in order to avoid an accident. You sound your horn. The other driver toots back and makes a rude gesture. If you are quick-tempered, you have already responded in kind. If not, this is the time to choose how to respond. You can become angry, thinking all kinds of destructive thoughts which you fling in the other driver's direction. If you become stressed, there will be little you can do to relieve it. If you shout and swear this may not take away your feelings of frustration; it may rather make you feel even more stressed.

Such strategies for coping are poor because they do nothing to help or improve the situation. With practice, you could choose more constructively. You could register the driver's bad behaviour, but realize that an input of negative energy from you will only make the situation worse. You could ignore it or you could choose to act positively. You might start by taking a deep breath and control your breathing. Then surround the other driver with pink energy (the colour of love), going with the thought that he or she needs healing to relieve the stress evident in his or her behaviour and to become more aware of the needs and feelings of others.

Your controlled breathing and positive thought process will calm you down and send a very constructive energy into the situation. It will pay dividends because like begets like.

This illustration could be extended and applied to many everyday situations which so often end up in frustration and distress. It is a healing strategy which extends mere coping to keeping your own power throughout. You are then in a position to improve a situation.

LIKE ATTRACTS LIKE

The mind has a powerful effect on the aura. Because like attracts like, the state of your energy field will attract people and events which are of a similar kind. So, if you want to 'have a nice day', you will need to have a nice mind which thinks nice thoughts. The choice is yours.

On the subtle levels energies accumulate in thought forms. There are aggregations of thought about all kinds of fear, anxiety, lack of worth, self-denigration, hate, jealousy, anger, and so on. There are also thought forms about joy, love, compassion, friendship, respect and admiration.

Once a pattern of thought is established in the mind, it will begin to attract a similar thought form. How many times have you felt bad about yourself as you mull over some of your weak points? Before long, negative thought forms have drawn close. You begin to feel worse. As the mind picks up the thought forms you are plunged even deeper into a fit of depression. What may have begun as an appraisal of some action on your part, may end up as a feeling that you might just as well not be on the planet for all the good you are doing. This is the insidious effect of negative thinking.

You have experienced this chain of events, without realizing the destructive role which thought forms have been playing in your experience. Think back to the last time it happened and resolve to be alert to the process from now on. If the process is recognized in time the train of negative thinking can be stopped and the thought forms withdraw. If not they continue to approach the aura until it is saturated in negativity.

But in just the same way, the laws of this process can be applied to produce positive outcomes. Positive thoughts attract more positive thought forms. Just a small effort to see a situation or ourselves in a positive light can set the process in motion to our lasting benefit. The more we exercise our ability to choose, the quicker the process works. So a lifetime of negative thinking will take a little practice to change, but it can be done.

We have to realize that, through the network of consciousness, every cell in our body is aware of our thoughts and responds to their energy. All negative thoughts have a negative effect on the body at the deepest, cellular level. Our negative emotions have a similar impact. These energies, coupled with their effect on the systems of the body, will sooner or later manifest as ill health for they are states of energy imbalance.

But all positive energies affect the levels of our being in a harmonious way, and manifest in the physical body as good health.

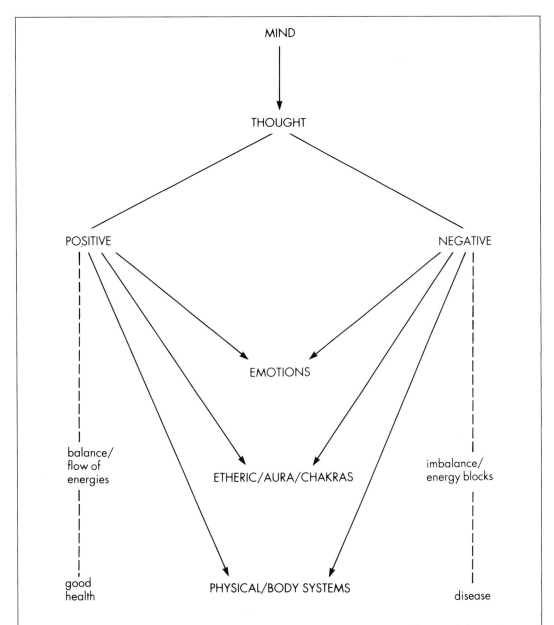

Fig. 23 Mind, emotions and health. The direct and indirect effects of thought. Energy entering the chakras on the etheric level is directed to the physical via the endocrine glands, blood system and nervous system. All systems and levels seek to balance and will compensate to bring this about.

SETTING YOUR OWN HOUSE IN ORDER

Healers can do much to help people identify how their thoughts and feelings are affecting them and to reprogram thinking patterns where necessary. But first you need to set your own house in order. How much do you know about your own ways of thinking? The next exercise will help you look at the way you think.

EXERCISE 35: Identifying Thought Patterns

○ Give yourself time and space to review the way you consider four different issues about which you feel strongly and about which you feel angry, emotional or disturbed in some way.

○ Write down these issues as concisely as possible.

○ Take each issue in turn. What do you think about them? Write down as many of your thoughts without analysing them. You will end up with four lists of thoughts.

○ Look at your four lists carefully. Have you been honest with yourself? If not repeat the exercise. Then sum up your four lists of thoughts. Does a pattern of thinking emerge and, if so, what is the pattern saying to you? How could your thought patterns affect your behaviour and your health?

○ When you feel you have answered these questions as well as you can, decide whether you are satisfied with what you have found out. If not, decide on a course of positive action.

○ Try the exercise with a partner and compare notes.

You may now be considering whether your emotions are working for or against you. Use the next exercise to gain clarity about the way the energies of feeling operate in your life. As before, give yourself time and space to work with the exercise. It will show whether you have constructive or destructive emotional aims.

EXERCISE 36: Looking at Emotions

○ Think about two recent situations where you have felt emotionally uncomfortable. Take them one by one.

○ Concentrate on the first situation and allow yourself to relax into it. See if you can get in touch with the feelings you had at the time. What happened when those feelings surfaced? Make a note of how you behaved. Was the result constructive or destructive?

○ See if you can recall feeling like that before and whether you behaved in the same way that time.

○ Move on to the second situation and note how you felt, how you behaved and whether the outcome of your behaviour was positive or negative.

○ Now look at the two patterns and see if you can understand where your feelings come from and if you could have behaved in a different way. Ask yourself how you can restore your emotional balance next time.

PROTECTING YOURSELF FROM NEGATIVE ENERGIES

Other people's anxiety, fear, anger, distress, etc. may all be absorbed into your solar plexus chakra so that you feel at least a degree of some disturbance. This accounts for the rapidity with which a crowd may become upset, violent or fearful.

Sometimes we are the target for other people's negative thoughts and emotions. These are powerful energies which we should avoid absorbing. Equally, we could be in a situation such as a meeting or a crowd where these kinds of energies are moving about. Being sensitive means that you can absorb them easily. But you can use your sensitivity as a positive attribute by being aware of what is happening and taking appropriate precautions.

The solar plexus chakra is the main point of entry for emotional and mental energies. When these are negative, the chakra needs to be protected. It is

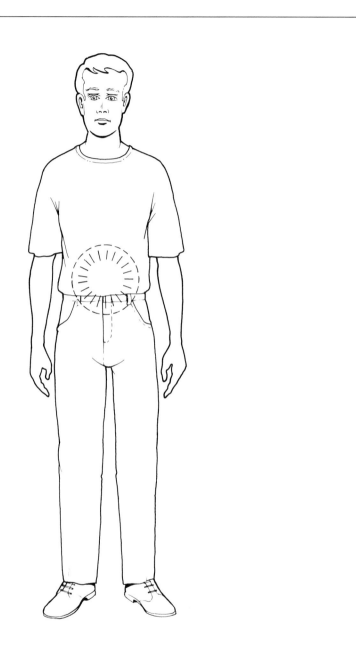

Fig. 24 The Solar Disc. Visualizing a disc of golden light covering the solar plexus chakra.

common to see people clutch something to their stomach when under emotional or mental attack or when in the presence of such conflict. This is the instinctive urge to protect the solar plexus which women are usually quicker to respond to than men. This urge is the correct response. Healers and all other sensitive people should use the following simple exercise as a protective 'cushion' for the solar plexus.

EXERCISE 37: The Solar Disc

○ To prevent the entry of any negative energies into the solar plexus chakra, visualize a golden disc of light covering it. Put the disc in place as soon as you enter an emotional atmosphere or when any negative thoughts are being expressed in your presence (Fig. 24).

When you are feeling in an emotional state yourself, you lose a great deal of energy. You can prevent this by putting the *Solar Disc* in place. But remember that you must then deal with the energies you are generating, if possible by giving expression to them via the throat chakra. This can be done by blowing, sighing, or even singing, until you feel you have released the pressure of emotional energy, thus avoiding damaging words or actions.

Once you have taken the appropriate precautions you can use your awareness to pour positive energies into difficult situations, thereby helping others as well as yourself. The energy of white or pale blue light tends to bring peace to an atmosphere, green light brings balance and pink light allows love energy to change thoughts and feelings, for the better.

It is worth remembering that often the discomfort you feel in the presence of others is simply due to the incompatibility between your energy field and theirs. As the chakras become involved in processing the incompatible energies, you sense this as discomfort. When this happens, either relax and allow the full spectrum of energy to enter your system and become balanced with it, or take the precautionary measure of using the *Solar Disc*.

RESPONDING POSITIVELY TO CHANGE

All healing involves change of some kind. In Rachel's case, change was a pressure which she felt coming from outside herself. The healer's task is to help the patient get in touch with what has to be changed, as well as how to respond to change itself.

In Deepak's case, the catalyst for change was inside him. He was an intelligent young man in his early twenties who had done very well at school. He had no problems passing the first stage of his accountancy exams and he had the full support of his parents. It seemed that his future was assured. But, after a brilliant first year in the office, Deepak had an emotional breakdown. He spent some months in psychotherapy and then went back to the accountant's office. As the time for the next exams drew nearer he became more and more distressed. His doctor said Deepak was suffering from acute anxiety and prescribed tranquillizers.

When he came for healing, Deepak had given up the medication, but he could not work. During the first year in the office, he realized he had often felt that he was doing the wrong thing, but he did not know why. He wanted a good career and he wanted to use his talents to get on in life. As he got in touch with his deeper feelings about his career choice, the true cause of his anxiety was revealed.

He had chosen the wrong job, but thought that in his case it was the only way forward. He really wanted to work with children, to be a teacher. The thought that made him sick with worry was that he had made the wrong choice and there was no way out. He would never get another grant to study something else and his parents would be disappointed. Most of all he feared the changes that would have to be made. He tried to comfort himself with the thought that accountancy really did make the best use of his abilities and that he would earn far less as a teacher.

Deepak had blocks in his solar plexus, heart and throat chakras. His fear and anxiety were centred in the solar plexus. His great fear of change meant that he had closed himself off from the promptings of his heart centre and could not express the truth of his heart's desire.

By working with these blocks in further sessions, Deepak was able to address his fear of change and listen to his inner voice. This enabled him to work out a satisfactory new career plan. His breakdown had been a breakthrough.

THE HEALTH EQUATION

When the soul is prevented from doing what it came here to do, the central theme of our lives is missing. But no matter what we do to anchor our life in materialism, our soul will not give up its struggle to make us see the light. It will find ways to exert tremendous pressure on us to change, even though change is what we so often fear.

The conditioned mind is alerted to the soul's pressure and does all it can to resist the call for change. After all, it can only envisage what it already knows and fears what it does not know. The personality panics, fearing what it interprets as disintegration if the demands of the soul are carried out. It does not stop to realize that the soul can only express itself *through* the personality, it is simply asking for this channel of expression to be opened to it.

Sometimes the pressure exerted from the soul level is so strong that we experience great discomfort mentally, emotionally or even physically. The refusal or inability to respond to the inner call for reconnection to spiritual reality can finally trigger a breakdown, as happened in Deepak's case.

As he worked with his fear of change he also found his way back to his inner Self. This enabled him to restore balance to the mental and emotional levels and bring health to the physical body. Deepak had to develop a new trust in himself and realize that when the Self is allowed full expression, harmony on all levels is the natural outcome.

When this happens, the wishes of the personality become the same as the soul's purpose. We are at one with ourselves and our actions express this harmony. The challenges which life may bring are addressed in a constructive way. The by-product is health and wellbeing. This is the health equation:

FULL EXPRESSION OF THE SOUL	=	ALL LEVELS IN BALANCE	=	HEALTH AND WELLBEING

In dealing with a life issue, a patient may choose to present only one part of the equation for healing. But during the restoration process, because of their dynamic relationship, healing works with all parts of the health equation. This means that healers can work with people to support them as they bring about both internal and external changes.

8

First Steps in Self-Healing

T he day you understand that you are in charge of your body, and take responsibility for your own health, is the day when you truly empower yourself. This may include a reassessment of your life, looking again at what is most important to you and what your priorities need to be. You will need to identify what causes you distress and what you can do about these causes. You will need to understand the effects of your thoughts and emotions and how much you are in control of them. Much of this you will already have begun to do with the exercises contained in the last two chapters.

REVIEWING THE PATTERN OF YOUR HEALTH

When you review your experiences as far back as you can, a pattern emerges of what you may call a healthy or an unhealthy life. To accept responsibility for your health, you need to understand what your own part in it has been. A first step is to link in with your body and have a dialogue about the pattern of your health to date.

EXERCISE 38: The Lessons of Ill Health

○ Think back over the years to the times when you were sick or out of sorts. Go back as far as you can.

○ Make a list of all the illnesses and mishaps you have suffered and list the people you can remember who cared for you at the time, or those who helped you get through.

○ See if there is a pattern to these times in your life and what energy centres they might be linked to. With hindsight, decide if these illnesses or mishaps were talking to you, stopping you, guiding you or showing you something. How did you respond at the time? For example, did you ignore the messages or signals or did you act on them?

○ Decide what part they have played in your personal development. Perhaps you are only learning now what certain conditions were teaching you. Thank your body for the experience and learning it has given you. Send out a thank you to all the carers and people who were there when you needed them. And remember your body has brought you through all these times.

REVITALIZING THE SYSTEM

As you have found from previous exercises, it is possible for you to become more aware of your body, to listen to what it has to say and to become more involved in the body's healing process. The work in this chapter gives you more practical support to enhance your new attitude of empowering yourself.

We are surrounded by the energies of the universal energy field, though we are not often aware of them. From a previous position of unconscious processor, you can consciously work with the energies to bring balance and healing into your life and into the lives of those around you.

Before beginning any process of rebalancing or revitalizing, it is necessary to clear the mixture of energies that are already present in the system.

EXERCISE 39: Clearing the Energy Field

○ Stand relaxed with the feet flat on the floor, a shoulder-width apart. Let the arms hang loosely. Breathe normally, through the nose.

○ Now imagine you are standing under a waterfall of silver light (Fig. 25). Allow this light to wash over you. Allow it to take away any incompatible energies which may be sticking close to your body.

○ Now see the silver light flowing through your aura, your own energy field, clearing away all the negative energies you have picked up during the day which you do not need.

○ Finally, allow the silver waterfall to stream through your body from head to feet. Visualize your body filling up with the silver light. Then let it flow out via all the orifices of your body, your fingertips and toes. Continue the process until you feel thoroughly cleansed inside.

    Now you may see beautiful colours entering of their own accord. This is a sign that your body and aura are cleared. Note the sensations of clearing and the sensations of being cleansed.

○ Breathe in and fill your body with white light, or choose a colour which you intuitively feel you need. Visualize that the waterfall of silver light has changed to this colour. Let it pour into you and breathe it in, but this time do not let it wash away. See the light completely filling you. (This exercise may be carried out lying down.)

In our daily dealings with other people, we cannot always avoid absorbing various energies from them into our own energy field. Some may be beneficial, but others are not. We also absorb energies from buildings, places, even the chairs and seats we sit on. Our thoughts and emotions add further energy components to the aura.

    Energies are absorbed according to the level of our development so that any healer or sensitive person will absorb much in one day. It is necessary therefore to clear the energy field to ensure sound sleep and to prepare us for the following day.

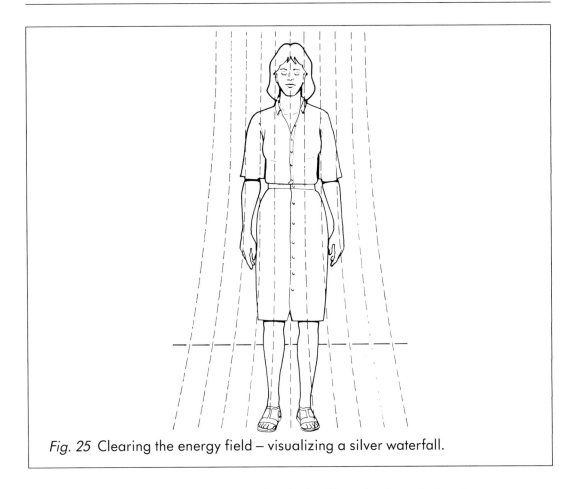

Fig. 25 Clearing the energy field – visualizing a silver waterfall.

The next exercise also clears the aura, but it should not be done during the hours of darkness.

EXERCISE 40: The Rainbow Bath

○ Relax the body, either standing or lying down.

○ Breathe in and visualize white light settling on the top of the head. Watch as it changes to a deep pink.

○ Now allow the light to flow down through you on the out-breath.

○ Repeat six more times, allowing the white light to change to orange, yellow, green, blue, indigo, and violet in turn.

This exercise clears and balances the aura. Since working with colour opens the chakras it should be done *before* any closing down exercise.

Clearing exercises may be followed by Exercise 30: *The Sphere of Protection* (Chapter 5). It should always be remembered that none of these exercises precludes a prayer for protection to your Guardian Angel, God or the Source of Love, or to those forces which you feel are looking after you. However, people who are channelling energies, such as healers, will wish to take responsibility for their actions as part of their soul's growth and maturity. If you are going to encourage others to take responsibility you will need to develop that same sense of responsibility to yourself and your work with the energies.

MAINTAINING YOUR ENERGY LEVELS

As well as the imbalances brought about by the effects of mind and/or emotions, there are other sources of energy imbalance of which we need to be aware.

How often do you go out shopping or mix with crowds only to find when you get home that you are completely drained of energy? This is because energy tends to bring itself into a state of balance. You may set off feeling full of vitality. Being a sensitive person, your chakras are always a little more open than average. Along comes someone low in energy. Just like a sponge they unconsciously absorb as much as they can as they move past your highly charged aura (Fig. 26).

After a few more people have topped themselves up in this way you may begin to feel quite tired. Perhaps you are surprised that you feel like this when you felt so full of energy at the start of the day; by mid-afternoon you need a good rest.

As a sensitive person, you must take control of this situation. Give your energy when *you* want to. When you feel people drawing on your energy, as you will by developing your sensitivity, offer up a prayer asking to be a channel for the energy that people need. In this way energy can flow through you to be used by others, without your own reserves being depleted.

Even though people will unconsciously draw on your energy in the normal course of events, you must not allow yourself to become depleted. There are simple ways of topping yourself up when you feel your reserves are low.

There may be times when you need the raw energies of the planet. These are life-sustaining at a basic survival level and should be drawn in when the system has become run down.

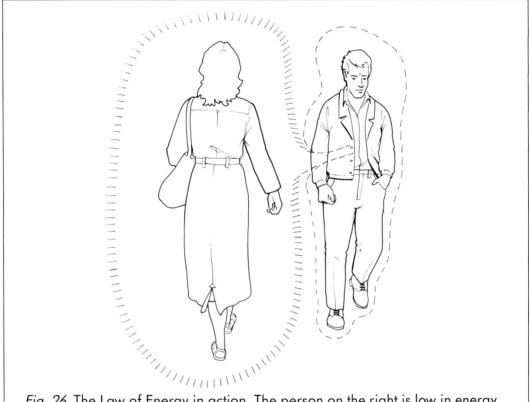

Fig. 26 The Law of Energy in action. The person on the right is low in energy and draws energy from the healer on the left as they pass in the street.

EXERCISE 41: Breathing in Earth Energy

○ Take off your shoes and sit comfortably with your feet flat on the floor and the hands on the thighs, palms upward.

○ Regulate the breath until it is slow, gentle and rhythmic. (As in all breathing exercises, breathe in and out through the nose unless the instructions say otherwise.)

○ As you breathe, visualize your feet making a good contact with the ground. Enjoy this feeling of contact with the ground.

○ Now breathe in, as if through the soles of the feet. Visualize the breath entering them as energy.

   (If you are unable to sit in this position through disablement, visualize the energy entering the base chakra.)

○ After three breaths, see the energy as a deep red/pink light. With each in-breath, draw this energy up your legs and into the rest of your body.

○ Keep breathing gently in this way until you feel fully energized.

The red energy can be used to energize the pelvis and legs and to assist in balancing all conditions in these parts of the body. You may like to try the exercise standing.

Follow this exercise by breathing in vitality energy as described below. Vitality energy comes to us from the sun and the cosmic sun. It is essential to our wellbeing.

EXERCISE 42: Breathing in Vitality Energy – Orange

○ Sit as before and make sure you are well connected with the planet (grounded).

○ This time focus on the sacral chakra.

○ Breathe a bright orange light into this centre. Let it first fill the area around the chakra and then keep breathing in this energy until it fills the whole body.

This energy energizes and balances all the organs and systems of the sacral region, including the lower back. It is particularly useful for women. It nourishes the organs of reproduction and helps with menstrual problems and related conditions.

EXERCISE 43: Breathing in Vitality Energy – Yellow

Vitality energy enters the etheric body at a finer rate of vibration through the solar plexus chakra.

○ Just as in the previous exercise, co-ordinate your breathing to breathe in this energy as a golden yellow light. First allow it to fill the solar plexus region and then gradually to fill the rest of your body.

This powerful source of vitality energizes all the digestive organs in the region and the associated systems. It vitalizes all other organs which may have become depleted and strengthens the etheric and astral bodies.

EXERCISE 44: Breathing in Vitality Energy – Pink

When the nervous system needs invigorating, a particular part of the vitality energy spectrum should be visualized. This has the colour pink. It is a great tonic – balancing and strengthening the system. Healers, carers and other therapists should never allow the level of this energy to drop too low.

○ Use the breathing techniques above to visualize a vibrant pink light entering the solar plexus chakra. Keep breathing this in until the whole of your body is filled with pink light.

When you are in touch with your own energy levels, you can select which of the above exercises you need to focus on at any particular time. Vitality energy can be given out to help others via the solar plexus chakra, but to avoid the loss of this energy against your will, visualize the Solar Disc (Exercise 37, Chapter 7), in place. If you wish to give vitality energy to another, make sure that in your mind's eye you remove the disc.

By practising the breathing exercises above, you have recharged your energy field. You have also cleared, balanced and strengthened it. Now you can take a further step to create a powerful aura which will draw other positive energy patterns to you. This is the creation and use of affirmations.

AFFIRMATIONS AS HEALING TOOLS

An affirmation is a phrase in the form of a message to the personality. It is a very powerful healing tool that can reprogram the destructive messages of the conditioned mind. By working on the source of these negative programmes, which are identified as trapped energies in, or between, the chakras, you can change the messages of the conditioned mind from self-doubt and self-loathing to those which are self-enhancing, life-supporting energies of security, value and love.

Affirmations are simple and effective ways to back up such work, to help a person regain power and restore energy balance. By linking with the heart chakra to create an affirmation, you can receive guidance on how to develop a certain quality or deal with a particular circumstance.

Your Higher Self knows what is holding you back and knows the exact wording of the affirmation you need. When you repeat your affirmation at the beginning and end of the day, you reprogram your mind and change your energy field in a positive way.

During healing programmes, patients have gained enormous benefit from using their own simple, creative phrases. I include some here as examples.

○ Sheila was working to correct a pattern of fear which had been absorbed through a violent father. Her first affirmation was: *'I know only love.'*

○ Andy was in the process of addressing the impact of a possessive, manipulative mother on his life. His affirmation was: *'It's safe to be me.'*

○ Louise had a long way to go in loving herself and accepting that she could change. One of her affirmations was: *'Loving myself makes me whole.'*

○ Lawrence, dealing with a lifetime of rejection which had stunted his growth in many ways, devised the affirmation: *'I am ready to grow.'*

EXERCISE 45: Creating Positive Affirmations

In previous exercises you looked at some of your thought patterns and some of your emotional patterns. These may have revealed areas of your conditioning which you would like to change. When you think about recent situations they may show you how your conditioning tape affects you in a negative way. You want to change your patterns.

○ Write down what your pattern is in a few words. Underneath write: 'I AM GOING TO CHANGE THIS AND I CAN CHANGE THIS.'

○ Now sit comfortably and relax. Take three full breaths then breathe normally. Let your mind focus on the heart chakra.

○ Think back to the pattern you identified in words. See the phrase you wrote underneath it.

○ Ask your heart centre to help you find one or more affirmations (positive statements) which you can use to change the pattern and the negative program. Wait calmly and patiently. When the 'still small voice' gives you the instruction you will recognize it as genuine.

○ When the instruction is complete, thank your heart chakra and visualize it gently closing up a little.

○ Take your time coming back to normal consciousness. Make sure you can feel your feet. Make a note of your affirmations and/or instructions. You now have a powerful phrase which, through daily repetition, will help you to change patterns and attitudes for the better.

Use the affirmation-discovery technique as often as you need it. Remember, the affirmations from your own heart are exactly right for you at this time. Keep a record of all your affirmations. It will serve as a useful guide to your development and will enable you to assess how you have brought about change since you started to use your affirmations.

Working with the heart chakra is a simple and lovely way to find out about positive thinking. It gives the mind a rest from having to 'come up with the right answer' and allows the heart to gently guide the mind instead. You will find it of great value to you and your patients.

RELAXING AND REFRESHING THE SYSTEM

The wisdom of the heart chakra can also be used to balance your body energies to relax and refresh the system. The following exercise can be done anywhere as long as you have a place to lie down.

EXERCISE 46: Balancing Body Energies for Relaxation

○ Loosen the clothing and undo any constriction around the neck. Lie down in a firm, comfortable place with the head supported if possible. The legs should be a little apart with the arms by the sides of the body.

○ Breathe deeply three times, letting go of tension on the out-breath. Breathe normally and let go of the body. Focus on the heart chakra with the eyes open.

○ Remain relaxed but alert, not allowing yourself to drift off. Let the body find its own position. Alertness is essential so that the body can speak to you as it gently finds its own balance. Notice how areas of tension relax. Some body parts may move slightly. Maintain your gentle focus on the heart chakra.

○ After about 15 minutes the body's energy system has become balanced. When this occurs, a tingling sensation or feeling of internal lightness may be sensed all over the body. Lie in this position for as long as you feel the need.

○ You will feel refreshed. Before getting up, give thanks for the body's ability to refresh itself in this way.

We continue the focus on balancing energies with a breathing exercise, well known to yoga practitioners as **Alternate Nostril Breathing**.

EXERCISE 47: The Balancing Breath

○ Sit in a comfortable position. Make sure that your back and neck are straight with the head held erect but relaxed. Do Full Breath Breathing three times.

○ Apply the first two fingers of the right hand to the side of the right nostril and press gently to close it (see below). Breathe in through the left nostril slowly and normally. Hold this breath for a count of three.

○ Transfer the first two fingers of the right hand (you can change to your left hand if you prefer) to the side of the left nostril to close it. Breathe out through the right nostril slowly and normally. Count three.

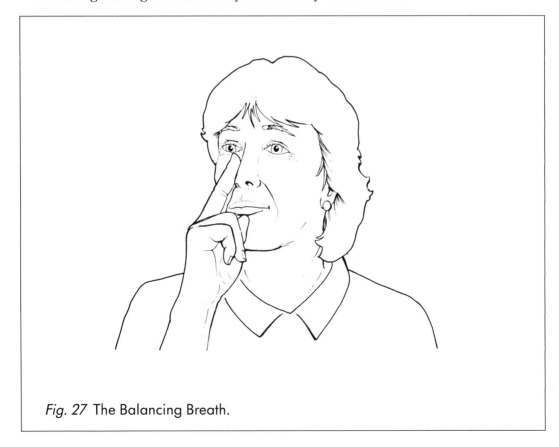

Fig. 27 The Balancing Breath.

○ Breathe in through the right nostril. Hold this breath for a count of three. As you hold your breath, transfer your fingers to the right nostril and breathe out. This completes one breathing cycle.

○ Do the cycle six times, slowly and gently. Then sit quietly for a few moments, being aware of the balance of energies in your body. Again, give thanks. The attitude of thankfulness after practising any exercise enhances its effects and sends a positive affirmation to the mind.

These first steps in self-healing have harnessed the power of the mind in a very positive way. In the next chapter, the human love of musing and daydreaming is focused in further techniques for self-healing.

9

Self-Healing,
Visualization
and Meditation

The mind is good at thinking up negative scenarios and the results are usually negative. But when the same power is harnessed to a positive aim you can use your ability to envision, or visualize, to great advantage. It just takes practice.

POSITIVE FUNCTIONS OF VISUALIZATION

Three very useful functions of visualization can be incorporated in your self-healing programme. The first function is to bring about *mental* relaxation. Here a peaceful scene is built up in the imagination which relaxes the mind and enhances bodily relaxation. Once you have carried out the following visualization exercise you will be able to use the technique to create a mental relaxation of your own whenever you need it.

EXERCISE 48: Visualization for Mental Relaxation

○ Sit or lie down in a comfortable position. Take three deep breaths and let go of any tension or anxieties with the out-breath. Relax your body. Let your mind settle peacefully.

○ Visualize a place you can go to where you can be totally at peace. Perhaps your mind will show you a place you already know. If not, visualize a peaceful place such as an empty beach, a forest clearing or a mountain side.

○ See your peaceful place in all its detail. See the forms and the colours. Look around you. Take in this scene of peace as you breathe slowly and gently.

○ Go for a short walk in your peaceful place. Enjoy everything you see and sense in other ways.

○ When you feel like it, sit down. Look around you again, slowly taking in the whole scene.

○ Now sit or lie down comfortably and be at peace. Stay in this place for as long as you need to and have time for.

○ When you feel ready, come back to where your body is, slowly and gently. Make sure you can feel your feet. Make a note of everything you felt and observed.

The next exercise takes the theme of mental relaxation a stage further. It will be most useful to record the exercise first, giving yourself time on the tape to carry out the instructions, or get a partner to read it slowly to you.

EXERCISE 49: Visualization – The Peaceful Garden

○ Sit or lie down in a comfortable position. Take three deep breaths and let go of any tension or anxieties with the out-breath. Relax your body and let your mind settle peacefully. Allow your mind to follow the visual exercise and allow your senses to engage in the process freely.

○ You are walking down a country lane at an easy pace. The sun is shining. There is a slight breeze which you can feel on your face. As you walk along you feel totally at one with things, at one with this country lane, with the air, with the sun, with your body. Your footsteps are light on the ground. Your body feels light and fresh inside.

○ You look to your left and see a horse grazing in a field. It is a picture of peace. You look to your right and notice some beautiful trees. Their presence is full of peace. You are at one with the horse, the trees and the field.

○ Ahead of you is a gateway which is inviting. You open the gate and see a path leading to a beautiful garden. You go up the path to the garden, noticing the flowers and shrubs as you pass.

○ There is a seat for you to sit on. As you sit down you notice the beautiful flowers nearby. You breathe in their scent. Birds are singing sweetly. The sun shines down on you as you breathe deeply and gently. Bees and other insects busy themselves about the garden. You feel at one with this place. Breathe in the peace of nature.

○ Stay here as long as you need to or have time for. When you feel it is time to come back, walk through the garden, down the path to the gate. Close the gate after you. Walk back down the lane, taking your time. Note the trees and the horse on your return. Give thanks to all that you see as you pass by. It is important that you come back exactly the same way as you first went.

○ Come back to where your body is sitting or lying. Make sure you can feel your feet. Make a note of any feelings or impressions you would like to record.

The visualizations above are a pattern you can follow to relax the mind. Use your imagination to create your own relaxing visualizations. Remember to include elements of peace and harmony in your scene. Any music which speaks to you of peace and harmony can be played softly in the background to further enrich the exercise.

VISUALIZATION TO OBTAIN GUIDANCE

The second function of visualization is to create a situation where you can obtain information, guidance, reassurance, where you can get help in problem solving, or where you can receive answers to important questions. This aspect of visualization is sometimes known as creative imagery. It is useful to distinguish it from other forms of visualization, for it is a method of using the technique to link with your inner guidance.

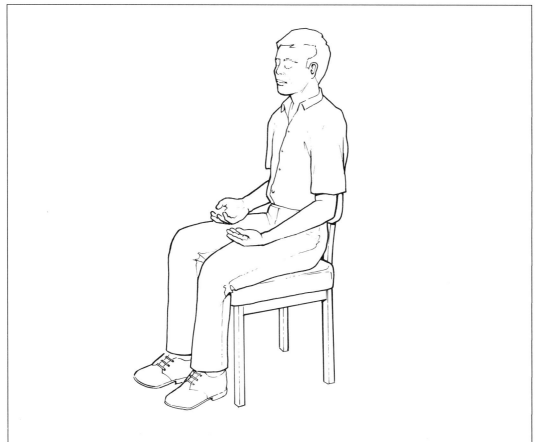

Fig. 28 The sitting position – for use in the exercises and when sitting for visualization or meditation when the sensitivity of the palms is needed.

EXERCISE 50: Using Creative Imagery

For the purpose of the exercise we will assume that you need some guidance on an issue you would like to address. You are going to use the technique to link up with the wisdom of the Higher Self so honour this with your attitude to the exercise.

○ Sit comfortably, with your feet flat on the floor and your hands resting palms up, on your thighs (Fig. 28). Relax the elbows. Relax the body and let the shoulders drop. Take three deep breaths then breathe normally. In your mind's eye you are setting off to a place where you will receive the guidance you need.

○ You see yourself walking along a road. The atmosphere is calm and peaceful. You feel light and optimistic within yourself. You are making your way to a special house. You see the house and recognize it by its appearance. The house has a welcoming feel, as if it is inviting you in. Go up to the front door which is open.

○ Inside you find yourself in a well-lit hallway which has some doors leading off it. You look at the doors. On one there is a label which says: 'Guidance. Please Enter.' Inside this room you will meet a wise person who will help you with your problem. Enter the room and wait patiently to see what happens.

○ When you have received what you need thank the wise person and close the door behind you. Leave the house carefully, noting as much as you can about it. Retrace your steps and return to your seat.

○ Give yourself time to absorb the experience before you gently 'come back'. Make sure you can feel your feet by moving your toes. Rub your hands together. Now make a note of the experience in as much detail as you can recall. Note down what you saw in the room as well as the house. Everything you see and experience is a clue to what you need.

  Perhaps you need further clarification, more information. Perhaps you have now thought of something else you would like to ask. You can always return to that room and ask for what you need. Just go back there in the same way as before.

Be prepared for the unexpected. Sometimes the material you need may be in a book or some other form. It may be just a simple message which you need to think about. People working with this exercise have reported that sometimes the 'wise person' does not take human form. Relax and allow your inner guidance to take over and show you the material in the way that is right for you.

Once you have become familiar with the format of these visualizations, you can use it to create images and situations for whatever purpose you require.

VISUALIZATION FOR HEALING

Harnessing the mind to healing visualizations can be a powerful therapeutic technique. It is a way of creating a visual form of affirmation and can be used in conjunction with one. The application of the technique can be as wide-ranging as you need it to be.

You have already seen in previous exercises how the network of consciousness allows you to contact any part or parts of your body that you wish. You have also discovered that the body responds to your communication with it in unexpected ways. The body has innate healing potential which will operate at all times unless we intervene in some way, such as via a negative mental message. This potential is a function of the balancing force in all the living cells of your body. If something is damaged, the cells will immediately set about repairing the damage.

You can co-operate with this process by using constructive visualizations and you will find that your body's response to them is extremely positive. You can use the following exercises for yourself or to teach someone else these self-healing techniques.

EXERCISE 51: Visualization for Self-Healing

This exercise can be used when you have had an accident or an operation and you wish to enhance your body's potential to heal.

○ Settle yourself as comfortably as you can and relax the body and mind. Breathe gently and normally.

○ Now allow your mind to focus on the injured part and send it loving thoughts. See the cells of the organs and tissues all being activated to carry out the healing as quickly as possible. See the blood bringing all the nourishing materials that the cells need to do their work.

○ If you feel impressed to flood the area with a colour, see the light covering the area, aiding the processes involved.

○ Continue with this visualization for as long as you wish. Let your intuition guide you to add anything else that is required. Let the injured part tell you when the healing is complete. Give thanks for the healing.

If necessary, repeat the visualization. Remember your attitude – not one of anxiety but of taking control. You are bringing in extra help to join your body in the healing process. Make sure your thoughts are linked to this process in a positive way.

HEALING DAMAGED SITUATIONS

Sometimes situations or attitudes need healing. For example, you may have had an argument or difference of opinion with someone which has left you both estranged. You are sorry about this. It is non-productive, destructive and helps neither of you. You would like to heal the situation, but you are wondering how to apply the knowledge you have about visualization and healing.

When Eric had a row with his wife and regretted it, he was in the same position. He was unable to finish his breakfast. He picked up his case and stormed out of the house without saying goodbye. He was going to be away on a business trip for the next two days. As he drove to the station, he felt awful about the row. He regretted his harsh words, not kissing his wife, and wanted to do something about it. In the station foyer he tried unsuccessfully to reach his wife by telephone. He had learned a visualization technique on a workshop and thought he might as well give it a try.

Sitting in the train, he visualized the link between himself and his wife and was shown a pink cord that was overstretched and frayed. In his visualization he repaired the link, using pink and gold light.

That afternoon he was called from his meeting to take a phone call. It was his wife. As they spoke to each other, he felt as if the rift had been healed.

There are many ways of healing damaged situations and the visualization exercise that follows is a possible way to work.

EXERCISE 52: Visualization for Healing Situations

In your visualization, see the situation in terms of a condition which needs healing and approach it in this way. There is no need to go back over what has already happened. Take the situation as it is *now*.

○ In your mind's eye see the other person. Tell them how sorry you are about things and that you are going to repair the damage with their help. Wait to see if they reply and accept whatever they say.

○ Now see the situation in symbolic form like Eric did. You can include yourself and the people involved if you wish. What sort of healing does the situation seem to need?

○ Does it need to be cleared first? If so, flood your symbol with silver light until it is cleared.

○ If the situation needs some love energy, see your symbol flooded with a deep pink light.

○ If it needs protection or strengthening, see your symbol flooded or enclosed with a golden light.

○ Finally, see the people involved smiling and united again. You have now done what you can at a distance. Hand the situation over to higher forces and let it go.

Be prepared for your inner guidance to add its own input to your visualization. In this second exercise the healing begins on a subtle level. You can use visualization in this way to 'prepare the ground' in advance. Note how your inner work changes the situation and in what way this happens.

Once you have used visualization for self-healing and experienced its effectiveness, you will be confident that for every condition that needs healing there is a visualization which you can create to help in the healing process.

MEDITATION – LINKING WITH THE HIGHER SELF

Where visualization uses the mind and the imagination for creative and self-healing purposes, the main purpose of meditation is to link with the Higher Self and the spiritual Source. This can only take place once the mind is still. All effective meditation techniques lead to this calming of the mind. In doing so, meditation allows the personality to make contact with the soul, providing a channel for soul expression. As you saw in Chapter 7, balance and harmony return once reconnection with your soul's mission has taken place. Meditation is thus one of the great healing techniques.

The mind alone cannot know the Self any more than it can know God or the Source. Hence the perennial problem of defining these truths. The mind's conditioning stands in the way of our linking with the Self. It therefore needs to be controlled, purified (in the sense of changing its focus from ego to soul) and finally transcended. Meditation is transcendental when it takes us beyond the limitations of mind, beyond thought, to an encounter with who we really are – the spiritual Self. This is the purpose and goal of meditation.

In the meditative state, the mind relaxes and the electrical activity of the brain's cerebral cortex moves out of the rhythm of everyday consciousness (beta rhythm). It assumes a new rhythm close to that of the sleep state (delta rhythm) or the state between sleep and waking, known as alpha rhythm.

The bodily processes under the control of the autonomic nervous system, such as breathing and heartbeat, slow down considerably. This allows our consciousness to move away from the physical to the subtle levels and ultimately to connect with Soul consciousness. This is experienced as a state of bliss by most meditators.

Apart from its physical benefits, meditation has been shown to be effective in stress release and is now an element in stress management and relaxation programmes. These positive effects act on the levels of mind and emotion to release stored negative and other unwanted energies. As we have already seen, repressed emotional and mental material may be stored in any part of the physical body and in the chakras. Meditation has the power to unlock these energies and bring renewed energy flow. Such releases of energy are quite normal and nothing to be alarmed about.

Meditators also report an increase in vitality, the curing of a range of physical conditions and a return to balance, lightness and wellbeing. This is due to the fact that meditation with a spiritual goal will transform the impulses which agitate the mind.

THE THREE STAGES OF MEDITATION

In the meditative state we are wholly conscious, but the mind is as still as possible. If prayer can be described as a 'talking' mode, meditation is a 'listening' mode. In this sense, the meditator does not carry on a dialogue but sits calmly and patiently. The most important aspect of this exercise is to be in the state rather than to expect some sort of outcome or benefit. Meditation is a state of being and not a state of expectation.

It is helpful to think of meditation as having three stages:

The first is *concentration* – finding a suitable focus for the mind.

Once the mind is comfortably focused you can move to the second stage, *contemplation*. This happens when the flow of concentration is uninterrupted and the focus unfolds itself of its own volition. At this stage the mind is still involved, but it is gradually becoming less active as other thoughts and distractions are simply allowed to pass through. This is a position of great strength and stillness and many healing benefits are obtained during this stage.

With practice, the mind is totally calmed and the link with soul consciousness is made. This third stage is known in yoga as *samadhi*, the blissful state of oneness. It is the true meditative state.

During healing, advanced spiritual healers enter a very similar state and it seems they are able to communicate or transfer this special state of mind to the patient. Researchers, such as C. M. Cade in the UK, have shown that this phenomenon also takes place during distant healing. Work with healers in the USA, such as Olga Worrall, confirms Cade's findings (see Further Reading).

TECHNIQUES LEADING TO THE MEDITATIVE STATE

There are many techniques which can still the mind and lead to the meditative state.

Visualization is a simple and common method where imagery provides the focus and subject for contemplation. When the mind finally relaxes, the third stage may be entered. For example, the technique could take you to that peaceful place where you are totally relaxed and calm so that the mind gradually becomes stilled.

Chanting, aloud or internally, or **sounds made with instruments**, can act as powerful focuses.

A photo, diagram, picture or symbol may be the starting point of a visual focusing of attention.

Many religions have evolved methods of contemplation which may or may not lead to meditation, according to whether the intention is to still the mind. Some of these methods have led to confusion over meaning. For example, if you contemplate a text, mull over its implications, and so on, you are not entering the third stage of meditation because the mind is still active. If, however, your focus on the text leads to a point where you stop contemplating and simply wait, you may well move into the meditative state.

ESTABLISHING A RITUAL FOR MEDITATION

Some people need a ritual to get them in the right mood for meditation. Anything which tells the mind that this is what is on your agenda is going to be useful. Once you have mastered a technique, you will be able to meditate anywhere and at any time, no matter what is going on around you. Until then, do whatever helps you to create the mood.

Choose a Regular Time.   Dawn and dusk are particularly good because the world around us seems to enter into a special tranquillity at these times. More important is to give the mind notice that at such and such a time you are going to meditate.

Choose a Regular Place.   If possible this should be set aside for meditation. It should be kept clean and fresh. You might like to keep a candle there, even a little shrine. Lighting a candle, dedicating it, dedicating yourself and your work, prayers, lighting incense – all these are signals to the mind that you want it to co-operate with you and honour this sacred time and space.

Sit Comfortably.   Sit cross-legged, or in the lotus position if you can, or in a chair. It is important to be comfortable, with the back straight and the hands resting on the thighs. If sitting in a chair, the feet should be flat on the floor. The elbows and shoulders should be relaxed with the head held erect (Fig. 28).

It has not been proved that the lotus position is the most effective position for meditation, though it is the preferred position in the East for cultural reasons. An attitude of joy in just sitting, in just being, without expectation, is essential to true meditation.

In China and Japan the meditation position is known as 'sitting like a mountain'. This gives the right feeling of solidity and stillness with the body well connected to the ground and the mind reaching to the heavens. When you sit, having this image of yourself will be very helpful to your practice.

For the healer, meditation is a spiritual act and a spiritual discipline. It puts us in touch with the Source of healing energies. It puts us in touch with the network of consciousness, linking us to all beings. Even five minutes of meditation is five minutes when we treat ourselves to being at one with all things.

A simple meditation follows which leads on from the visualization earlier in the chapter. Having mastered it, you can devise your own visualizations to lead you into meditation.

EXERCISE 53: Visualization Leading to Meditation

○ Carry out the whole of *The Peaceful Garden* visualization up to the point of sitting in the garden. Do not look around the garden anymore. Do not follow the progress of birds etc. Just sit and wait patiently.

○ Remain alert and aware of just sitting. Allow yourself to 'be' in the garden. Start with five minutes and then build up to half an hour.

○ Return to normal consciousness gently and become aware of your feet. Make sure you can feel them and the ground beneath you.

○ Make a note of your experience of this meditation in any way you wish.

BREATHING – A POWERFUL FOCUS

Many religions, especially Buddhism, use the act of breathing as a powerful focus for meditation. Here is a meditation exercise which is very good for beginners.

EXERCISE 54: Meditation – Following the Breath

○ Sit in your meditation position. Let your body sway gently from side to side three times to reach a point of balance.

○ Relax the body, especially the neck and shoulders. Check that no other part is clenched or tight.

○ Breathe in slowly and naturally six times. Follow your breathing. Note how you breathe, then pause, and how you breathe out. Follow your normal breathing.

○ If the mind wanders off bring it gently back to your breathing.

○ Carry out this exercise for five minutes. When your focus is strong extend to eight or 10 minutes. Over the weeks, build this up to 20 or 30 minutes.

DEALING WITH DISTRACTIONS

Whatever meditation technique you find appropriate, in the early stages you may be acutely aware of distractions. If you anticipate this you won't be so unsettled by them when they happen. For example, you will be aware of your body. It may itch or develop a pain. Acknowledge these feelings, then let them go. They are simply distractions of the mind. You will become aware of sounds. Just be aware of them and let them go. Thoughts will come into your mind. Just let them pass through without hanging on to them or following where they lead. Let them go.

Note things which distract you. Note how the mind complains and tries to interest you in other things. Think of the mind as a horse which needs to be trained. You are the trainer. Treat your mind kindly but firmly. Now you are ready to try some more meditation techniques.

EXERCISE 55: Meditation – The Heart Chakra

○ Prepare for meditation as in the previous exercise. Breathe normally. Focus the mind in the heart centre. Your spiritual ideal resides here. Without expectation, know you are entering your sacred space to be with your Higher Self.

○ With this focus, watch your internal screen and wait. Be still and at peace. Allow all thoughts to enter without resisting or censoring them. Regard them with detachment as if you are watching a flowing stream. Do the same with pain or any other sensation. Let all these forms of energy pass through. You are a strong and tranquil mountain. All these things may pass through you unhindered. If the mind wanders, bring it back to the heart centre and carry on.

○ When your sitting is ended, come back into your body calmly and deliberately. Become aware of your surroundings, your feet and your contact with the ground. Breathe the air. Give thanks. Allow yourself to return to material consciousness.

Start with a focus of five minutes and build up to 20 or 30 minutes a session.

EXERCISE 56: Meditation – Chanting Om

In India, OM is a sacred Sanskrit syllable which is said to be the cosmic sound giving rise to all creation. It is the 'word' as in St. John's gospel. It is intoned by opening the mouth and letting 'A' emerge from the back of the throat. The sound moves forward through 'U' until you gradually close the lips on 'M', which becomes an extended hum. You can see that OM encompasses all sounds which can be made by the human voice.

○ Sit in your meditation position and chant the sound syllable OM either aloud or internally. Focus on the whole of the sound from beginning to end.

○ Once you are proficient in following the OM, you can co-ordinate your chant with a focus in the brow chakra which it activates. To do this, visualize the sound emerging from the brow chakra and also being absorbed by the brow chakra. This is an advanced meditation technique.

MEDITATING TO UNBLOCK AND OPEN THE CHAKRAS

Once you have become at ease with the meditation exercises given above you might like to try another advanced technique recommended by the avatar, Sathya Sai Baba (see Glossary). The energies of this meditation work on many levels at the same time. They help to unblock and open the chakras, especially the heart, throat and brow chakras.

EXERCISE 57: The Candle Flame Meditation

○ Settle yourself in your meditation position with a candle and matches within reach in front of you. Light the candle and dedicate it to your spiritual ideal.

○ Say any prayers of dedication, thanks and protection which come to you.

○ Balance your body and your breathing.

○ Now look at the flame of the candle carefully. Notice the aura of light around the flame. Close your eyes and see the whole of the flame and its light within your brow chakra. See it illuminating this centre and gently opening it.

○ Slowly let the flame move down into the heart chakra. See it bathing the heart chakra with its light and gently opening it. All darkness has left the heart. Now, the light grows until it fills the whole of your chest, at the same time it spreads into the shoulders and down your arms. It spreads further to fill the abdomen, pelvis and your legs.

○ Now the flame slowly rises up into the throat chakra where it illuminates this centre and gently opens it. It moves to the mouth as the light of truth and trust. Slowly it rises into the head and fills the head with light. It shines from the eyes and ears. All darkness has left the mind. The light in the heart glows more strongly and from your fully illumined body it shines out and around you.

○ Let the light fill the room in which you are sitting. Let it spread further to surround your loved ones, relatives, friends, colleagues, your enemies and rivals, strangers and finally all beings and the planet itself. Allow the light to fill and illuminate everything.

○ Wait in this light. Be in this light. This is the light of the soul, the light of the Source of all things, of all energy. Thank your spiritual ideal for the light. Come back in the same way as in the previous meditation exercises.

HEALING A SPECIFIC CONDITION

By carrying out the exercises given in the book so far, allowing the energies to work at the various levels (by relaxing and letting go!), you will have embarked on a powerful and effective programme of self-healing. To deal with a specific condition carry out the following self-healing exercise.

EXERCISE 58: Self-Healing

○ Lie down comfortably or sit in your meditation position. Do some full breath breathing and wholly relax the body.

○ Attune yourself to the Source of healing energies by prayer, affirmation or whatever statements seem to lift you to this level. Ask for healing to be sent to you in whatever way is appropriate. Remain as open and relaxed as possible so that you can experience whatever form the healing might take.

○ When you feel the healing is over, give thanks. Carry out the closing down and protection exercises you have already learned.

Attunement and the act of healing are covered in more detail later in the book. You may wish to include some of these techniques in your self-healing at a later date. Try to work through the book in the order given since each exercise builds on the knowledge and practice already gained in earlier chapters.

Self-healing is the direction of healing energies towards your own condition, whether that is physical, emotional, mental or spiritual. But at a deeper level it involves a total commitment to aligning your personality with the Higher Self. In doing so, you are made aware of what needs to be healed.

The exercises in the next two chapters, dealing with daily issues, will support and complement your self-healing programme.

10

Your Personal Programme

Another day begins. Will you tune into the energies of life or will you remain unaware of them? The choice is yours. Your first thoughts and acts of the day can help set the tone (the energy pattern) for the rest of it. They will create a certain vibration within you and a certain energy field around you.

STARTING YOUR DAY

When you wake up, you move into your waking state of consciousness. You may have come from a dream state, an out-of-body state, or a deep sleep state – the different levels of being which you have been experiencing.

There are many ways of being woken. When you wake naturally, you are usually at the end of a sleep cycle of about 90 minutes and you come back to the waking state in a few moments.

But this is not always the case. When you are woken before the end of a sleep cycle – the alarm goes off or you hear a sudden noise or feel a sudden movement – you may experience a number of feelings ranging from irritability to extreme drowsiness.

You need to realize that you have left your sleep at a stage which is not the best time for you. You may have left something unresolved such as an unfinished dream. Worse, you may have been out of your body and had to hurriedly return, so that you feel confused or even angry.

Before getting out of bed, take a few moments to gather your thoughts and senses. If you have to set your alarm, next time give yourself a time allowance to centre yourself and carry out some of the exercises which follow.

STUDYING THE DREAM STATE

This is an important part of your life and, as Carl Jung recognized, it deserves as much study as the experiences of your waking life.

Take time to recall as much of your dreams as possible before getting up, before they have the chance to slip away. Make a note of them in your journal or in a book kept by your bedside for this purpose.

EXERCISE 59: Dream Recall

○ To recall a dream, either start at the end and work back, or at the beginning, trying to recall the sequence of events. Another way is to recall any significant part of a dream, gathering as much detail as possible, and then to work from this point until all of the dream has been collected.

○ The atmosphere and feel of a dream are as important as the events, and the best interpreter of your dreams is yourself. Decide what the dream is telling you and make your own interpretation.

○ If you feel upset due to an interrupted dream, tackle this straight away before negative thoughts and emotions have the chance to build up and take over. Centre yourself while still in bed and breathe slowly and deeply. Put one hand over your solar plexus, to soothe the upset feeling. Tell yourself that if the dream had an important message which you have missed, you will receive the message in another dream at another time.

○ Continue to breathe slowly and deeply, enjoying the calm this brings. Congratulate yourself on taking the initiative instead of letting negative thoughts and feelings build up. You are in control.

THE HEALING POWER OF DREAMS

One of the important functions of the dream is to heal. Material may be processed in a dream and this brings about healing. Very often people receive healing in the dream state, when they are more accessible to the energies. I have found that patients' dreams are a valuable part of their healing process.

Gordon's case is a typical report of direct healing while in the dream state. He initially came for spiritual healing because of a temporary loss of hearing. On his second visit, Gordon spoke about a dream which occurred the same night as his first healing session.

In the dream he saw himself standing quite calmly and relaxed. He watched in amazement as his head was tipped first towards his right shoulder and then to his left shoulder, as if his neck was made of rubber. What he described as 'gunge' seemed to pour from each ear. This action was repeated until the flow from his ears had ceased.

Gordon was having a powerful healing dream for the next morning he was awakened by birdsong. His hearing had returned.

BEING OUT OF THE BODY

It is perfectly natural to leave the body during sleep. We do this to experience other levels of existence and to meet up with people on these levels. It is very common, for example, to meet up with those who have passed over. If there is someone we need to talk to and this is not physically possible, we can meet them on the astral level. Sometimes we give healing or help others in some way and it is easier to do this when distance, for example, is no object. It is also common for healers to receive important teachings on this level.

All this is done through astral travelling – travelling on the subtle levels in our astral body. While we are out of our physical body, the life force keeps it 'alive' until our return.

For many people, out-of-body experience is not understood as part of their normal consciousness. The brain therefore interprets it in the only way it can – as a 'vivid dream'. Being out of the body is not confined to when we are asleep of course. As I have already described, this happens to healers in the normal course of events during a healing session and when doing distant healing. It is also very common for patients to leave their bodies during healing and this may be essential in some cases. This is why precautions must be taken to make sure both parties are grounded (back in their bodies) at the end of the session.

As with dreams, if out-of-body experiences have been interrupted, this is not serious. They can be returned to during the sleep state at another time. It is important, though, to be back in the physical body during the waking state, for obvious reasons. Take time to get properly back in your body.

EXERCISE 60: Getting Back in Your Body

○ Remain lying down and relax, breathing slowly and calmly. If you are feeling agitated, put one hand over the solar plexus.

○ Imagine you are out of the body looking down at it. Tell yourself that it is time to return now and move down towards it. Slip in at the crown of your head, feeling yourself easing gently and completely back into the physical.

○ Wiggle your toes. Push your feet against something and make sure you can feel them.

○ Gently move the rest of your body about then relax the muscles. If you still feel light-headed, give yourself a little more time.

THE HEALING POWER OF WATER

Water is not only the best medium for cleaning the physical body, if you are feeling out of balance, with things on your mind, water helps to clear the situation.

EXERCISE 61: Using Water to Clear Negativity

This exercise is ideally done under the shower where water acts like the clearing waterfall you practised in Chapter 8 (Exercise 39).

○ Let the flowing water clear away worries and anxieties from the day before and thoughts or memories which may have been causing you discomfort during the night.

○ Visualize them falling away from you in the glistening droplets.

Water will clear negative energies and restore balance to the body which has been affected by them. This is the unseen but vital function of the bath, shower or wash.

Washing is a process of cleansing, symbolic of an inner clearing, preparing for a fresh start. The same process can be entered into before you get ready to go out somewhere or to wash away the events of the day before going to bed.

If you have been in an argument, a tense or stressful situation, immersed in unpleasant vibrations of any kind, the healing and cleansing power of water can be used to clear these negative energies from within and around you.

Water which has been blessed and consecrated for ceremonial, ritual or cleansing purposes is purified and its vibrations quickened. Blessing is a way of increasing the power of a substance while at the same time giving thanks for it.

An exercise in the next chapter shows you how to charge water to make it into a tonic. Once you know how to do this you can drink your water tonic as a system cleanser. This is best done first thing in the morning.

GREETING THE DAY AND GIVING THANKS

Once ablutions are complete, if the weather is fine you can go outdoors to greet the day, though the following exercise is just as effective indoors.

EXERCISE 62: Greeting the Day

○ Face the east, the place of the rising sun and the dawning of the light. Even if the sun cannot be seen, it can be visualized in the mind's eye. Stand or sit and relax the body.

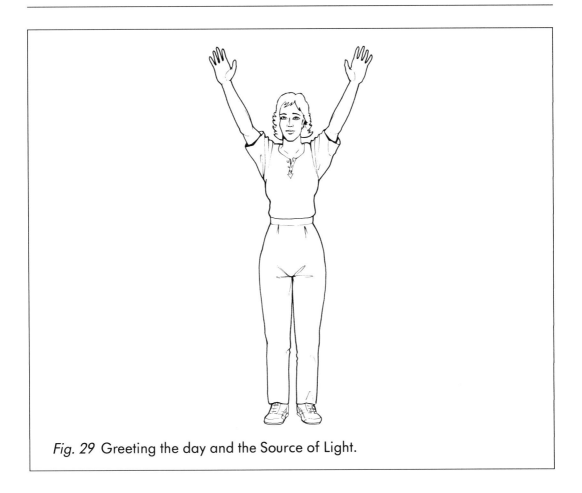

Fig. 29 Greeting the day and the Source of Light.

○ Give thanks for the previous night. Be aware of the source of energy within you.

○ As you face the sun, become aware of its golden rays beaming towards the planet, bathing everything in its energy. Feel your body fully connected to the Earth.

○ Now, as you breathe in slowly and deeply, raise your arms above your head in salutation (Fig. 29). Stretch up. This is the position of prayer. Give thanks for the day and greet the light. Give thanks to the sun for its nourishing energies. Feel the air around your body. Give thanks to the air. Breathe in deeply. Release the breath slowly, lowering your arms as you do so.

EXERCISE 63: Creating the Sphere of Love and Peace

○ Continue standing or sitting with your arms by your sides.

○ Breathe in again, visualizing that you are inhaling the light of the cosmic sun through the sacral and solar plexus chakras.

○ During the out-breath, allow the inhaled energy to fill all parts of your body. Keep breathing in the vitality energy until you feel totally energized.

○ Now visualize that you are breathing in spiritual energy through the crown chakra. In your mind's eye, see this energy becoming a deep pink colour as it enters you. Breathe it in slowly and gently, filling up your entire body.

○ Breathe in the deep pink energy once more. On the out-breath send this energy of love to all beings in front of you. It may help you to say mentally: 'I give love to all beings before me.'

○ Breathe in again and on the out-breath send the energy of love to all beings behind you. Within you, say: 'I give love to all beings behind me.'

○ Allow it to flow out from you, over the place where you live and out over your country, extending as far as your imagination will allow.

○ Breathe in again and on the out-breath send the energy of love to the left of you. 'I give love to all beings to the left of me.'

○ Breathe in and on the out-breath send the energy of love to the right of you. 'I give love to all beings to the right of me.'

You have now created a circle of light and love which extends all around you.

○ Breathe in again and on the out-breath send the deep pink energy to all beings above you, entering and refreshing them as it passes through them. 'I give love to all beings above me.'

○ Breathe in once more and on the out-breath send the energy of love to all beings below you. 'I give love to all beings below me.' See the light extending far below and far above you. You have become the centre of a pink sphere of love which extends in all directions.

○ Now see planet Earth in your mind's eye, as if from space. See it enclosed in your sphere of pink love energy.

○ Enclose it with a second sphere of peace in the form of sky blue or white light. Finally, see the planet enclosed a third time in a sphere of golden light. This is a sphere of strength and protection. You have now enclosed the planet in three spheres of light (Fig. 30).

You may wish to send these energies to various parts of the planet which you feel need extra help. This is the time to do so. For example, if you know there is trouble in a certain place, see this area on the surface of the planet and bathe it in the twin energies of love and peace.

These energies are first absorbed at an etheric level which is greatly benefited. Then they are sent to the physical level of the planet where they give further benefit.

You may know of people, animals, plants or part of a landscape needing this help. Now is the time to direct these energies to where they are required.

Do not worry if you cannot see or visualize colour. As long as you are mentally directing the energy, the work will be done.

You are now in a very good state to do some meditation (see Chapter 9) to reinforce your creation of a positive energy pattern for the day. The contact with higher forces will allow you to be a channel for information and guidance for yourself or those whom you meet later on. It is the one exercise which truly centres you.

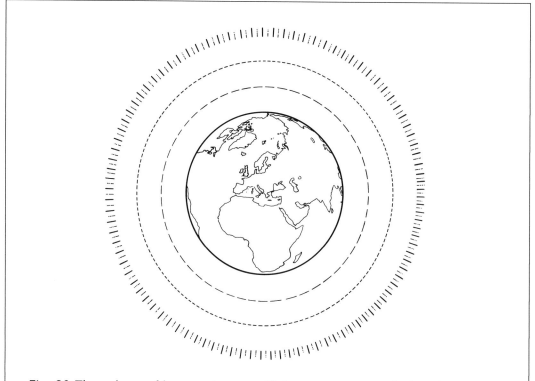

Fig. 30 The sphere of love and peace. Pink energy surrounds the planet. This is enclosed with the pure energy of peace. Finally, the planet and these energies are protected by an outer sphere of golden light.

POSITIVELY ENERGIZING YOUR FOOD

The calm, balanced state after meditation is ideal for preparing food. But worry about the day to come, the journey, your job, people you will have to deal with, things you have to do, generates negative energy which food will absorb. If you are preparing food for others, you owe it to them, as well as yourself, to be in a positive frame of mind. Breakfast, the first meal of the day, can be a time of celebration.

A grace or blessing helps you recall where your nourishment comes from. It may be said aloud to link all present in the thanksgiving and it also demonstrates the point to young children who are still learning about these matters. If you wish to give thanks mentally, your own words, sincerely meant, have the greatest power.

Your thanksgiving might begin with the Source of all nourishment and energy. Then give thanks to Mother Earth who has provided the physical sustenance. Then thank the plants and animals whose bodies go to make your food.

It is worth remembering that, when eating out, you often have no idea who has prepared your food or what state of mind they were in at the time. By asking for the food to be blessed, any negative vibrations in it will be cleared.

Food should be enjoyed. Your calm enjoyment sends encouraging thoughts to your body which can then make the best use of it through the process of digestion and assimilation.

POSITIVELY ENERGIZING YOUR WORKPLACE

To review the day ahead and prepare yourself for work, see it from your still centre. Know that if you ask for the help of the higher forces around you it will be given. Before you leave for work, or during the journey to it, you can fill the workplace with positive energy in the following way.

EXERCISE 64: Energizing Your Workplace

○ Sit or stand in a relaxed state.

○ Breathe in. On the out-breath visualize the workplace being bathed in healing light. Let the light go to every corner, illuminating every area of darkness or shadow. Sometimes this exercise takes effect quite quickly. By the time you get to work, the air may have become clear and light and other people may remark on this. They may even be laughing more than usual or seem more contented. So your work of spreading the light benefits your colleagues as well as yourself.

○ Sometimes your place of work needs the energy of a particular colour, just like you do. See the place in your mind's eye and ask it what it needs, or ask to be shown the colour. This is the colour you should fill the workplace with.

HEALING NEGATIVE RELATIONSHIPS

There always seems to be someone who is able to make life difficult for everybody else. This is partly because other people allow this to happen.

Someone who is causing you problems may be acting like this. But, if this is your way of seeing them, they only seem to be like this. They may be holding a mirror up to you so that you see a side of yourself you do not much care for.

They may be jealous or fearful of your abilities. They may be going through a hard time and need help. Try to discover the real reason for their difficult behaviour. Decide whether your perceptions are biased and see if others feel the same about this person. Frightened, unfriendly people need reassurance and compassion for they are actually suffering.

Very often it is possible to turn a situation around and realize that you may be the person to achieve this. Do they need a listening ear? Could you send distant healing? Do you know someone else who could help too? Decide how to act to heal the situation. Everyone is trying to deal with life in their own way and this may not be your way.

Remember the Solar Disc (Exercise 37, Chapter 7). No matter what vibrations other people are giving out, you can protect yourself from the negative effects of these by applying your new knowledge. Perhaps you would like to send healing to a situation or help certain people. The following two exercises use specific energies to heal and balance.

EXERCISE 65: Thinking Pink

The deep pink of love energy has profound healing effects and you can always surround a person or situation with this energy – by thinking pink. The nervous system is soothed and the etheric body strengthened by pink energy. It changes attitudes and thinking patterns from negative to positive and gives powerful help to anything that is bruised, torn or injured, whether this is a person or a situation.

○ Visualize a sphere of pink light around the subject. Co-ordinate the visualization with your breathing and send this energy on the out-breath. If it is difficult for you to see colour, visualize something pink like a bunch of pink roses or a pink balloon.

○ If you are going to a difficult meeting or an interview for a new job, project pink into the room beforehand. This will not, of course, make the meeting go *your* way, and you won't get the job if it is not right for you, but it will encourage an outcome which is best for all the parties concerned. It will also help to create a relaxed atmosphere of trust and confidence.

RESTORING BALANCE

It is no coincidence that people go off to the country when they need to find peace and balance. The green colours of the plant world supply these valuable vibrations. Breathe them in and always give thanks for the gift. Use the next exercise whenever you feel out of balance emotionally or mentally, such as when you feel upset. It can be used to help balance people, or a situation, as in the previous exercise.

EXERCISE 66: Thinking Green

○ Visualize green light being drawn down to the crown of the head. As you breathe in, this colour flows down over your head and body, and then flows out to fill your aura.

○ On the in-breath, say in your mind: 'I breathe in peace and balance.' On the out-breath, release the cause of your tension or upset state.

○ Now breathe the green light in through the crown chakra and let it fill your body. Say in your mind: 'I breathe in peace and balance.'

 The energy of green light may also be used to energize the organs in the chest, the heart and circulatory system. Breathe the green light into the heart chakra. Allow it to fill the heart chakra and then the physical body via the meridians and thymus gland. The lungs and bronchial tubes also benefit from this energy.

ENDING THE DAY WELL

And so you have made your way through the adventure of your day. Before you prepare for bed, take some moments to assess your day in a detached frame of mind. Tell yourself that you are going to look back over the day, not to praise or blame, but to see what has been achieved.

EXERCISE 67: Reviewing the Day

○ Sit or lie comfortably. Breathe normally and relax the body.

○ Think back to the morning. What was your mood like? What did you set out to achieve and did you achieve it? How did you react to things that happened or problems that occurred? How did you react to the good things in your day?

○ Now decide how you might react if there was a next time.

○ Many people may have crossed your path today. Did anyone stand out for any particular reason? Did anyone stand out as needing your help? How have you reacted to these people?

○ Ponder the role you played as you crossed other people's paths today.
    You are training to develop awareness of yourself and others as beings of light. Did you see the light of another person today? Were you really looking for it?

○ Having considered all these aspects of your day with a sense of detachment, simply let them go. The things of tomorrow will be dealt with tomorrow.

PREPARING FOR SLEEP

A routine of meditation and/or prayer will create the right atmosphere around you, and the right frame of mind for sound sleep and useful dreaming.

The next day really begins the night before. This is because your thoughts and feelings last thing at night, and the quality of your sleep, affect the day which follows – they are the energy base you will have to build on.

Before retiring to bed, check that you will be as physically comfortable as possible. You will not sleep well if you have given your mind too much to digest. Do you really want images of horror and distress stored in your mind at all, let alone last thing at night? Physical, emotional and mental indigestion means that your valuable dream time will be taken up with processing the agitation this causes on the etheric and astral levels.

Check that your mind and emotions are calm and do not attempt to sleep with an unresolved argument or with harsh words ringing in your ears. An apology or other peaceful overture, as appropriate, could be a small price to pay for an untroubled mind and a good night's sleep.

Emotional and mental turmoil ruins sleep. If you cannot sleep because of your disturbed thoughts, you are under stress. Waking in the night or following morning with the same thoughts on your mind as the day before is a sure sign of stress. Address the cause before it becomes a source of serious energy loss and imbalance.

Give thanks for your day. You have done what you can. Before finally going to sleep, carry out the clearing, closing down and protection exercises you now know. Look forward to your sleep. If you wish to remember your dreams, tell yourself that you will do this. Agree to be a channel for healing during the hours of sleep on condition that you will not awake feeling depleted of energy. Put yourself in the hands of the highest. Try smiling as the last thing you do, it is a great healer.

CONSOLIDATING YOUR WORK

The exercises you have practised so far provide you with a range of material from which you can design a daily or weekly programme for change, empowerment and personal development. Use the next exercise to formulate your programme and to decide how much you can include in it.

EXERCISE 68: Building Your Personal Programme

○ Find a quiet place and think about your day and how much time you can realistically give to this work. Make a note of how long and when you have this time available.

○ Look through the exercises and pick out those which you feel you would like to incorporate in a personal programme. List them in order of priority. Some exercises could be practised daily, others weekly. By comparing your time slots with what you would like to do you can build your initial plan.

○ Copy out your initial plan in your journal.

○ Work with this for a while before you make any changes. Make notes on how you get on with your programme. When you make changes, put a note giving the date and your reason for the change.

○ When you have extra time for yourself you might like to extend the programme. When time is pressing, look again at your priority list.

ASSESSING YOUR PROGRESS

You have come a long way since you started working with this book. Let's look at what has been accomplished. You have studied the causes of ill health and energy imbalance. You have equipped yourself with a range of proven techniques to clear, balance, strengthen and vitalize your energy system at all levels. You have begun a powerful realignment process which will bring about your own self-healing.

All this has been the essential groundwork to prepare for what may be the most important work on yourself as you offer your time, energy, experience and love to care for others. In the final part of this healing journey you will learn how to build upon your own abilities and use them as a healer.

11

Your Healing Hands

*S*ally *was looking very unhappy and complained of a bad headache. It was making her feel dizzy and sick, she said. Her mother was a healer and responded to Sally's request for help. After attuning herself, she went to put her hands on Sally's head but something stopped her. Instead she held them near her daughter's stomach and abdomen. Straight away she felt energy pouring into these areas as her hands grew hot.*

Sally shifted in the chair. 'I'm feeling better already. What are you doing?'

Her mother didn't answer but changed position and gently held Sally's head for a few minutes until she could no longer feel energy leaving her hands. She knew then that the healing was completed.

Sally smiled. 'Thank you. Don't tell me, it was that restaurant, wasn't it?'

The cause of the headache seemed to be a contaminated meal and instant attention had been needed where the action was!

SENSITIVITY AND INTUITION – HAND IN HAND

When you begin healing, your hands will lead you to the place where healing energy is needed. They have a subtle sensing apparatus which is sensitive to energy flow and imbalance. This sensing mechanism is activated and guided by the power of intuition.

As you allow the sensitivity of your hands to work in tandem with your intuition they will prove, with practice, to be a guide and helper whom you can trust. The listening, trusting attitude has been emphasized throughout this book and, if you have practised the exercises, you will have become thoroughly used to this by now.

Your hands will have their own healing signal which will tell you when they are ready to work, for example a tingling sensation or heat. When the work is complete the tingling or heat stops. During the healing they may feel hot or cold, heavy or light, and they may even tremble. These are other examples of how your hands may react to the energies which you are channelling.

The following exercises will deepen your awareness of your hands and the to and fro of energies which pass through them. This is the preparation stage for beginning your work as a healer.

EXERCISE 69: Sensing the Quality of Your Hands' Energies

○ Stand or sit comfortably. Take three full breaths to energize yourself.

○ Hold your hands up to about waist height, with the palms facing inwards, and the width of your body between them. Let the hands relax so that the fingers separate naturally. Notice what you sense.

○ Bring them together slowly, again noticing what you sense as you do so (Fig. 3, Chapter 1).

○ Try again with the hands stretched a little wider apart. This time be more aware of the energies. You could think of them like strands of elastic stretching from hand to hand.

○ Vary the distance between your hands. Turn them over. Move your hands together in different ways. Note the various sensations.

Now you are ready to work like this with another pair of hands.

EXERCISE 70: Sensing the Energies of a Partner's Hands

○ Stand opposite your partner. Hold your palms up at about chest height, to face your partner's palms. Let the hands relax so that the fingers separate naturally.

○ Slowly move your right palm to meet your partner's left palm. Then move your left palm to meet your partner's right palm. Gently pull your palms back towards you. Let your partner try these same movements.

○ Now both of you move both sets of palms together. Slowly pull them back again. Notice what you sense in this exercise. Was it different from sensing your own energies? Discuss the sensations with your partner.

Your hands are receptive to energies, as you have just experienced. Let's see what happens when you encourage this process with visualization.

EXERCISE 71: Breathing Energy into the Hands

○ Sit comfortably with your feet flat on the floor. Rest the hands on the thighs, palms up. Relax your elbows, the back of the neck and top of the shoulders. Close your eyes if this helps your concentration.

○ Focus on the centre of your palms. Visualize light beaming down into them and make a note of what you feel or sense.

○ Now visualize that you can 'breathe' this energy into your palms. As you see the energy beaming down, breathe in. On the in-breath the energy is absorbed into your hands. On the out-breath it fills your hands and arms (Fig. 31).

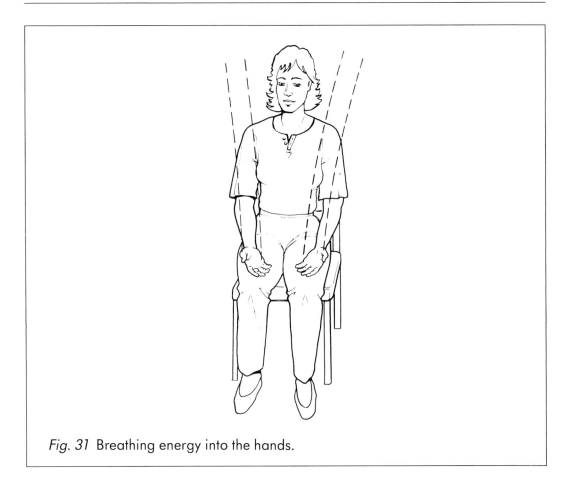

Fig. 31 Breathing energy into the hands.

Note your sensations and compare with the first part of the exercise. Follow this with the next exercise.

EXERCISE 72: Sending Out Energy from the Hands

○ Raise your hands to about chest height, with the palms facing away from the body.

○ Visualize that you can beam energy *out* from your palms. What do you sense?

○ Fill the hands with energy on the in-breath, send out the energy on the out-breath (Fig. 32).

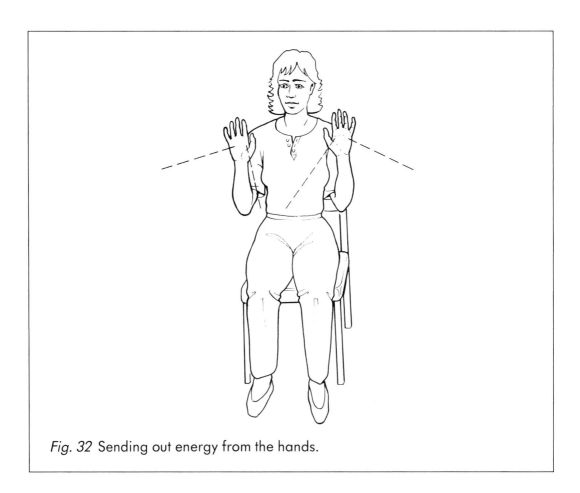

Fig. 32 Sending out energy from the hands.

EXERCISE 73: Sending Energy to a Partner

○ Sit opposite your partner, who should be sitting at least two yards away from you. Both of you hold your hands up about chest height with the palms facing outwards. Take three full breaths to energize yourself.

○ (Your partner should remain receptive.) Breathe in. On the out-breath send energy from your hands to the palms of your partner's hands. Repeat.

○ Now try beaming energy to your partner's hands by thought alone, without co-ordinating it with your breathing. Note all your own sensations.

○ Change round, with your partner carrying out each stage of the exercise. Again, note your sensations. What did it feel like receiving energy from your partner? Compare notes together.

CHANGING THE ENERGETIC PROPERTIES OF WATER

I was able to convince a sceptical dowser that a healer's hands can charge water – change its energetic properties. She dowsed a glass of water and then watched with surprise as her pendulum swung widely over the water after it had been charged. She told me it must be an excellent tonic and proceeded to quaff the whole glass!

EXERCISE 74: Charging Water

○ If you are in need of a healing tonic, fill a glass with water. Ideally this should be still spring water. Hold you palm over it, an inch or two from the surface (Fig. 33). What do you experience?

○ Ask for healing energy to be directed to the water. You may feel this energy being transmitted through you. If your palm tingles keep it there until the tingling stops – it is charging the water.

○ Once the water has been charged, drink it slowly, visualizing that you are sipping healing light. Make a note of your impressions. You may be aware of a faint colour, for example, or even a change in taste.

This exercise can be used to help someone else. Ask to be a channel for healing for them and charge the water in the same way.

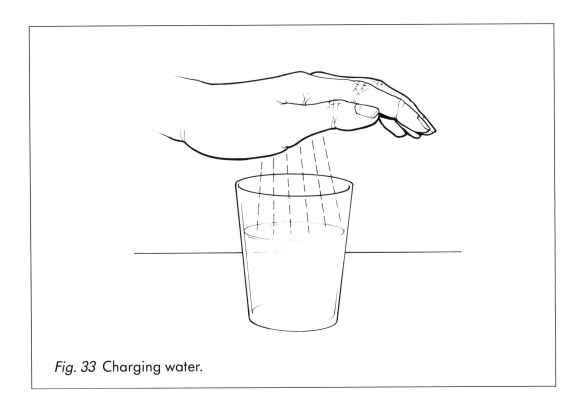

Fig. 33 Charging water.

SENSING OTHER NATURAL ENERGIES

All things are energy patterns. Living things are surrounded by an energy field or aura. Now you can experiment with the sensitivity of your hands to see if you can sense the aura of a plant. Start with a pot plant or a small plant outdoors.

EXERCISE 75: Sensing the Energy Field of a Plant

○ Hold your hands over a plant without touching it. Bring your hands
towards the plant slowly and gently until you feel its energies meeting
yours.

○ You are in contact with part of its aura. What does this feel like? Do not
project energy from your hands, but allow the plant to take energy from
you if it needs it (Fig. 34).

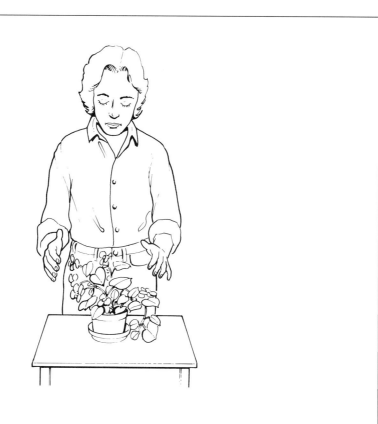

Fig. 34 Sensing the energies of a plant.

The next time you sense a plant needing energy, hold your hands over or near it and ask for healing to be channelled through you to help the plant.

These exercises show you what your hands are aware of and give you a preview of what they can do. When someone raises a hand to bless their food or to comfort another person, you can understand that this is no mere gesture when linked to a conscious intent.

Get in as much practice as you can in just sensing with your hands. The next time you feel pain and go to put your hand over the place that hurts, realize that you can direct healing to it. This is the fundamental use of the hands in hands-on healing.

ATTUNING TO THE SOURCE OF HEALING

Before Sally's mother put her hands on her daughter she attuned herself. This should be done before any healing work, whether hands-on or distant, even when charging water for someone. It is the first and vital step in opening yourself to be a channel for healing energies. The purpose of attunement is to link with the Source of healing and to thus raise your consciousness to the highest level possible. This not only prepares you for work but ensures that you *channel* energy without using up your own. Once you have practised the attunement exercise you will be able to attune in an instant, at any time and in any situation. Take your time and enjoy the feeling of being at one with the Source of healing.

EXERCISE 76: Attunement for Healing

○ Sit comfortably with your feet flat on the floor, and with your hands, palms up, on the thighs. Relax your elbows (Fig. 28, Chapter 9). Do three full breaths and relax the body. Be aware of your feet in contact with the ground.

○ Give thanks for the opportunity to be used as a channel for healing. Ask to be as pure a channel as possible. Ask for protection for yourself and your patients. Dedicate yourself and the work, asking for it to be blessed. Say any other prayers that you wish.

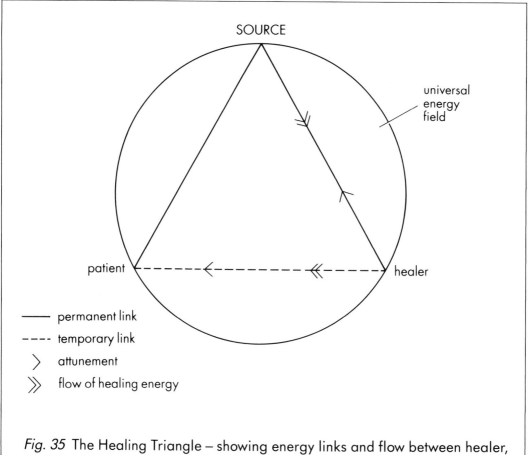

Fig. 35 The Healing Triangle – showing energy links and flow between healer, patient and the Source of healing energies.

○ If you have time, you can extend your attunement to create a peaceful, healing atmosphere. The energies of healing are energies of love and peace. Breathe in love and visualize it filling your body. You can visualize it as pink light. When you are totally filled with this energy, breathe in again and, on the out-breath, allow the love energy to surround you and fill the space where you are going to work.

○ Now breathe in peace and let it fill your body. You can visualize this as sky blue or white light. When you are filled with the energy of peace, breathe in again and fill the space around you with peace.

○ Sit for a few moments in the aura of love and peace which surrounds you and the workplace. This is the atmosphere you have created for your patients. They will notice it and they will benefit from it.

Once you have attuned, you have made your link with the Source of healing energies and you have created the first side of what I call *The Healing Triangle*. When you link with whom you wish to help this creates the second side. This is done by consciously linking to the Higher Self of the other person. In this way you activate the third side of the Healing Triangle, which is their own link with the Source. This powerful healing structure is a flow of energy, set in motion by unconditional love (Fig. 35).

Now you know how to properly attune, you should carry out this exercise before you do any healing work. You are a channel for healing energy which you can direct through your hands. Make the following exercise part of your self-healing programme.

EXERCISE 77: Using the Hands for Self-Healing

○ Sit or lie down comfortably and carry out attunement.

○ Having asked for healing to be channelled to help yourself, put your hands over the part of your body which needs healing.

○ Keep them there until the healing is complete (Fig. 36).

○ Give thanks and surround yourself with the golden light of protection. Visualize your hands being cleared of your condition by seeing them 'washed' in silver light.

DISTANT HEALING

As I described in the Introduction, I began to work seriously as a healer through distant healing (sometimes known as 'absent healing') and I would recommend it as the best way to get started. You will soon get a feel for the

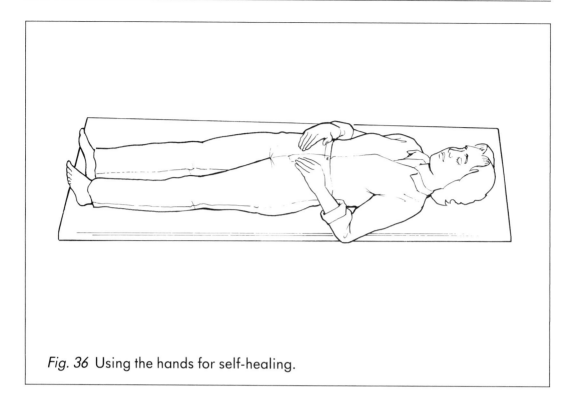

Fig. 36 Using the hands for self-healing.

work and be able to decide whether you actually enjoy it or not. You will start to understand what part your hands want to play in it and how effective you are when healing at a distance. It is a very good way of getting to know your own hands' healing signals.

In its simplest form, distant healing can be a prayer that healing will be sent to the person who needs it. The request should be made unconditionally so that the healing is directed where it is needed and not where we, with our limited knowledge, think it should be. In other words, we ask for *healing* for someone without limiting our request to something like: 'Please cure her cancer.' This honours the fact that a person is a spirit and not a body and that it is the spirit which dictates the healing force. It also honours the soul's evolutionary journey and deeper reason for a condition which we actually know nothing about.

If a person asks for distant healing for themselves for a specific condition, I still recommend that you send healing unconditionally.

The following exercise will get you started with distant healing. It is also very effective when carried out with a partner or group.

EXERCISE 78: Distant Healing

Choose a time when you will not be interrupted by callers. Disconnect your telephone or switch on the answerphone. Make sure you have your list of needy people, animals, situations, etc.

○ Attune yourself as described earlier. Light a candle and dedicate the light to your distant healing. Ask for protection. Give thanks that you have been given the opportunity to send out healing light.

○ Focus your mind on the heart chakra. If you have a spiritual ideal, such as a symbol or representation of the Source, for example, see this in your heart chakra.

○ As you inhale, visualize this centre filling with light. See your chest expanding with the light.

○ Now see this light extending from you to a place in front of you. (If you are working with a partner, sit opposite each other with a space in between. If you are part of a group, sit in a circle so that you enclose the light.) Once you are aware that the light has formed up in front of you realize that this is the light of healing. It is still there, even if you cannot 'see' it.

○ Now ask for your list of needy people to be put or held in the light. It will help to read the names out aloud, one by one. (Within a group each individual may offer names.) You may see these people or you may not. It is important that you know your mental intention, motivated by love, has put them in the light of healing (Fig. 37). This linkup forms the second and third sides of the Healing Triangle.

○ When your list is complete give thanks. As you blow out the candle you might like to think of *this* light being sent out to where it is needed – a strife-ridden place, an environment under threat, and so on.

○ This exercise could be followed by meditation. If not, do the closing down and protection exercises. (More distant healing techniques will be described later.)

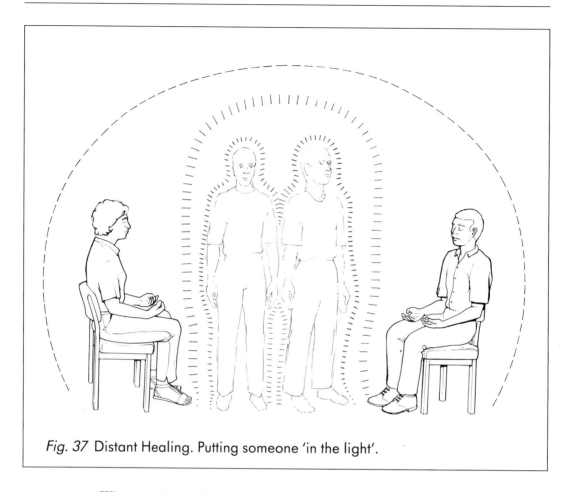

Fig. 37 Distant Healing. Putting someone 'in the light'.

When people ask for your help as a distant healer, ask them in return to let you know how they get on. Feedback is essential so that you have a way of monitoring what happens. Keep a note in your journal of healing progress or distant healing requests and any feedback you receive. Some healers work entirely in this way and find it as effective in most cases as 'hands-on' healing. It is the best way of working when people cannot travel, where people are confined for various reasons or where there is a mental or behavioural condition.

Sometimes a person would never go for healing, but a friend or relative wants to help them. This is not an intrusion if the distant healer asks for healing for that person in the usual way (without specifying the condition). It will then be up to the recipient, at a soul level, to decide how they will use the energies.

If that person does not use them, the energies will flow to where they can be used.

Healing energies come from the Source. This means that they originate *outside* the space/time frame of the physical and so are not governed by its laws until they enter this level. Thus they can travel to another person, at any distance, in an instant.

Once the soul becomes aware of the energies directed to it, interaction takes place from a soul level downwards. Sometimes energy will reach the physical instantly and bring about change. Sometimes energy will be needed on the subtle levels first and change will be seen on the physical more slowly. These things depend on the cause of the condition, the soul's journey and the state of readiness of a person. They may also depend on the balancing factor of *karma* (the law of cause and effect). This comes into operation when the soul decides to address imbalances created in past lives.

Spiritual healing honours a person as a spirit and does not see health as an isolated condition of the body. It also honours the body consciousness and seeks to co-operate with it, rather than to manipulate it.

WORKING HANDS-ON, FIRST STEPS

While you work as a distant healer you will be gaining confidence and learning a lot more about how healing works. Then the time will come when you feel ready to work directly with patients. Resist the temptation to go looking for them. Distant healing is effective healing and you can carry on with this while things unfold.

As your energy field develops, the law of attraction will come into operation and you will find people being directed to you in various ways, seeking your help. This is because you are the right person for the job, whether or not you have worked with the particular condition. The next chapter will explain in detail how to conduct a healing session.

If you live near a healing group such as an NFSH healing centre or spiritualist church (see Useful Addresses) this could be another way to get started. Each centre will have its own procedures for integrating you into the group, but here you will have the opportunity to work as a probationer alongside experienced healers. Healing centres and groups are the public face of the healing organizations they represent and tend to deal with a wide range of clients, which is ideal for new healers needing experience.

YOU NEED HANDS

When you start working with patients, one of the first things they will notice about you is your hands. You will need to be aware of them too, and keep them looking presentable. Notice what you usually subject your hands to.

You will need to wear gloves if they are going to get scratched, blistered or very grimy doing some chore.

If you cut your hand, put a plaster over the wound before you start your healing session.

Your hands must be in the best possible condition for they are the visible link between you and your patients.

It is time to join the ranks of the 'hand conscious.'

12

The Healing Session

When you intend to work with the public on a regular basis or take up healing as a profession, it is prudent to belong to one of the healing organizations (see Useful Addresses). Some organizations are attached to religious bodies while others, like the NFSH, are non-denominational.

The healing organization will register you as a healer once you have reached the required standard of proficiency, as well as keep you in touch with other healers and latest developments in the field. You will be insured as a spiritual healer as part of your membership fee, but you will not be covered for any other therapy which you may practise alongside spiritual healing unless you have separate insurance. This is a safeguard for the public and it encourages high standards of professionalism.

Your membership of a recognized healing organization also provides an assurance for your patients that you abide by a professional code of conduct. The Confederation of Healing Organizations (CHO), for example, has agreed a Code of Conduct with the medical profession, nurses, midwives, dentists and veterinary surgeons, which must be adhered to if you are a member of an organization which is affiliated to the CHO.

The NFSH encourages its members to learn the basics of first aid so that they know how to act if an emergency occurs during the patient's visit. This is unlikely to happen, but it is wise to be prepared.

PRACTICAL ADMINISTRATION

You will need to decide on your availability – how many hours you will be giving to healing. A treatment should continue for as long as healing energies are being directed to the patient, so that a complete session may last from at least 30 minutes to an hour.

You will need a telephone so that patients can book appointments in this way. Keep your diary nearby. Make sure you make a note of their name and telephone number. At the booking stage it is appropriate to say what your fee is per session. Some healers do not charge a fee, but are willing to accept 'donations' and, if this is the case with you, it should be made clear.

Have you decided to work from home, at a clinic, a centre or with a doctor?

Consider how your patients are going to find out about you. Will you advertise or will it be by word of mouth or referral?

You should allow time between sessions to make brief notes about your treatments. It would be more difficult at the end of the day to recall everything that occurred. It is essential to keep a record of your sessions, no matter how brief this may be, but respect your patient's confidentiality. A simple card index can be kept on which you note the date and time of the appointment and a few words describing the treatment given. Be aware of the security of your record system.

GENERAL PREPARATION

The day before you are to receive and work with your first hands-on patient, check the room where you will be working. It should be fresh, clean and tidy. On the day, flowers always give a special feel to a room.

Decide whether it is appropriate for your patient to use a chair or healing couch. A healing couch allows the healer easier access to the patient, but your choice should depend on the presented condition and what is going to be most comfortable for the patient.

If you want to use quiet, soothing music for relaxation, make sure that it is in place with your player in working order. Ideally, relaxation music should be unbroken and without sudden changes in tempo or volume. Does your player make a loud noise when it reaches the end of a cassette side? This could be upsetting for both you and your patient especially if you have entered a deep state of focus. You may find some people are distracted by music.

Certain household noises can be disturbing in the same way. Make sure the telephone is not within earshot, or disconnect it for the duration of your session.

Consider how you will accommodate other people. If patients arrive early, will they have somewhere to wait and will there be someone to open the door? Some patients bring other people with them. Will they be welcome to sit in on the session or will they be asked to go away and return later?

If the companion needs to wait in another room it is a good idea to have reading matter available, especially books and magazines containing articles about healing.

If you are going to work with patients of the opposite sex, you will both feel more comfortable if they bring a chaperone.

You will need to write down a few simple details about your patient so make sure materials are available for this. A box of tissues may be required.

Some patients need to use the toilet. Check that it is clean and that there are handwashing facilities also. Finally dedicate the healing room to the work.

This routine of preparation will help to put you in the right state for healing before the patient arrives, but the most important part of the preparation is your own attunement. This is your creative alignment of spirit, mind and body with the energies of healing. Attune yourself as suggested in the previous chapter.

MEETING YOUR PATIENT

Greet your patient with a smile. Show where coats may be hung and where the toilet is. Some people may have travelled long distances and a glass of water helps to settle and refresh them, especially in hot weather. Make your patient as comfortable as possible before you get down to obtaining a few personal details for your records.

As you talk together, you may start to receive impressions from the patient (as you did in the exercises of Chapter 2). Keep them to yourself and remain open minded. Ask whether the patient has already seen a doctor and how you can help. Say that you will do your best but, like any doctor, you cannot promise a cure.

It should be remembered that if you become aware that your patient is suffering from a notifiable or infectious disease, your patient must be advised to see a doctor immediately and not permitted to come into contact with other people. A list of notifiable and infectious diseases can be obtained from your doctor or health centre.

Give your assurance that what takes place in the healing session is strictly confidential. Your attitude should be optimistic, kind, receptive, empathetic, calm and confident at all times.

It is important to study factors in communication such as your tone of voice, the way you present yourself, your body language, any prejudices or strong views which you may have. You must be able to *listen* with interest and empathy and to express love and understanding in appropriate ways. Interrupting, finishing your patient's sentences and giving unasked for advice are not loving responses.

This is the time to put all other things aside, including whatever you may feel about your patient. Be there with your patient, for your patient.

PREPARING FOR HEALING

When you have a clear picture of your patient and the presented condition, you have completed the first part of the session. Ask if your patient has ever had spiritual healing before. If not, say a little about what you will be doing and how it works, so that your patient feels at ease.

Ask if your patient objects to being touched. For some people this can be very upsetting. Actual contact with the body is not necessary in healing, but it can be very comfortable in many situations. It is best not to touch the front of the body, where people are most vulnerable, and certainly not the genital area. For women, contact with the breasts may be considered an assault.

There is no need for the removal of clothes, except an outside coat. Some people like to remove their shoes and this should be encouraged, though it is not necessary.

Take note of the presented condition when you ask a patient to sit or lie down. During the healing, patients need to feel safe, whatever position they are in. If they do not feel safe it will be difficult for them to relax.

GROUNDING

Pay attention to your patient's body position. If s/he is sitting, the legs should be uncrossed with the feet flat on the floor. The hands should be unjoined and rest easily on the thighs with the elbows relaxed (see Fig. 28, Chapter 9). These precautions relate to grounding or earthing the healing energies circuit. When these energies enter the physical plane they are very similar to electromagnetic energy and have to be treated as such. For this reason, make sure that your feet are touching the ground at all times too.

If you patient is lying down, the legs should be slightly apart, with the arms at the sides of the body. Here grounding occurs because the patient's body is in contact with the healing couch, which is in contact with the ground.

As mentioned earlier, the chakras in the soles of the feet and base of the spine deal with our interaction with planetary energies at an etheric level. During healing, we also need to provide the correct physical connections wherever this is possible.

THE IMPORTANCE OF RELAXATION

Your patient may be tense or nervous, especially if s/he has never had healing before. Make sure that you relax the patient as fully as possible with the simple breathing and relaxation exercises you have already learned in Chapter 9.

ATTUNEMENT TO THE PATIENT

The second part of the attunement process reinforces the other sides of the Healing Triangle. Its purpose is to link with the patient and make her or him aware of this link. This in turn makes the patient more receptive to the healing and activates her or his own healing potential.

Explain to the patient that, if s/he is agreeable, you will do this by simply standing behind the patient and gently placing your hands on the shoulders (Fig. 38). As you do this, link with the patient at a soul level by mentally thanking her or him for this opportunity to work in this way and asking the soul to direct the healing. If the patient does not wish to be touched, you can attune by holding your hands just *above* the shoulders. Then proceed in the same way. A similar position can be assumed if the patient is lying down (Fig. 39).

This simple act enfolds the patient in the atmosphere of attunement which you have previously created.

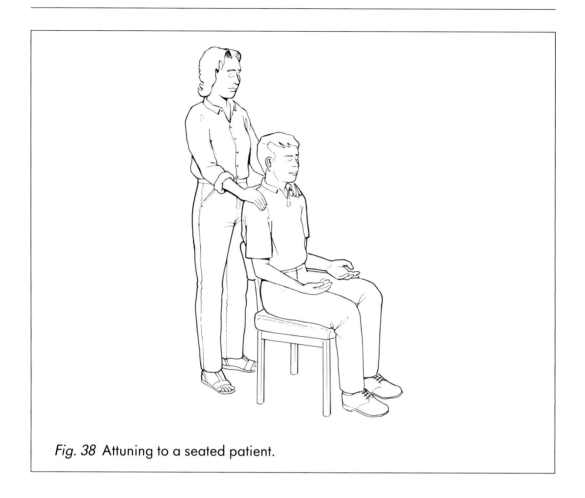

Fig. 38 Attuning to a seated patient.

THE ACT OF HEALING

Every healer is ultimately 'taught' through their own inner guidance (hence the importance of developing this link), but experience has shown that people find it helpful to have a sound, straightforward base on which to build. The healing method described in this chapter provides such a framework. Once you have mastered it, your own way of working can evolve from this in a natural way.

Since the patient directs the healing (through attunement), the healer does not decide the outcome. Healing comes when we are relaxed, allowing the heart to open and make the decisions at soul level. So relax, enjoy your work.

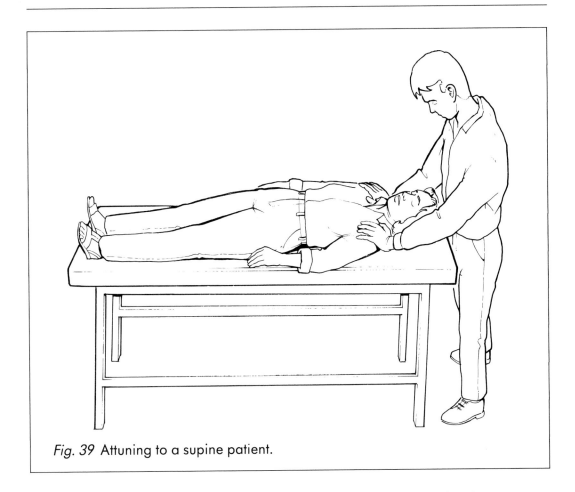

Fig. 39 Attuning to a supine patient.

The basic healing act can be divided into three 'scans' and their associated healing. A scan is where the hands are used as sensors to obtain energetic information about the patient – to monitor energy flow, energy imbalance, the need for healing input and so on. With practice the scan becomes an extremely sensitive and comprehensive technique whereby a great range of information can be accessed.

When treating a patient for the first time it is usually best to begin this way so that you have a complete picture of their energies right from the start.

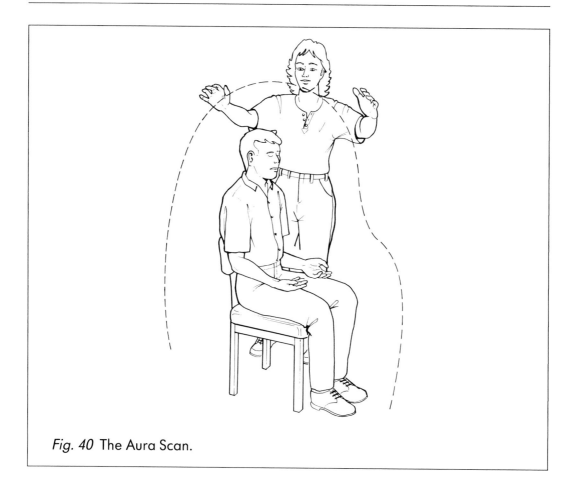

Fig. 40 The Aura Scan.

EXERCISE 79: The Aura Scan

In this first scan, the techniques you have learned earlier are developed to become a healing skill.

○ Move far enough from your patient so that you can extend your arms to sense their aura. Let your hands relax so that the fingers separate naturally. Start above the head and move slowly round and down to the feet. Note any changes or discrepancies in the shape and feel of the aura.

Be as open as you can to impressions which you may pick up (Fig. 40).

○ Note where you feel impressed to return to any part of the aura. This will be done after the three scans.

The aura scan can also be carried out on a patient who is lying down. Hold your hands above the body, then bring them down slowly until you sense the aura. Start at the head and make your way to the feet (Fig. 41). The total aura can be sensed in this way without asking the patient to turn over.

The aura scan is a way of sensing the subtle bodies of your patient. This provides useful background information to the condition which your patient is presenting.

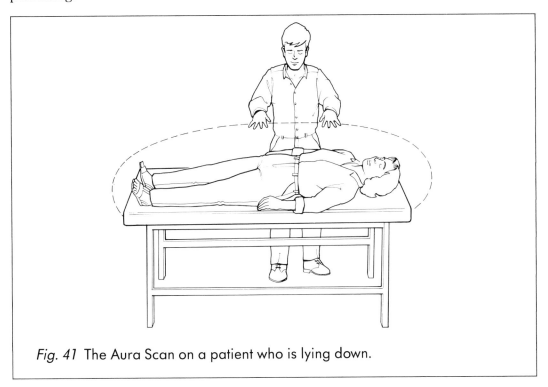

Fig. 41 The Aura Scan on a patient who is lying down.

Now we move into the etheric body to scan the energy system. This is your first opportunity to notice the links between the chakras. As you carry out the chakra scan you may sense blocks to the flow of energy either within the

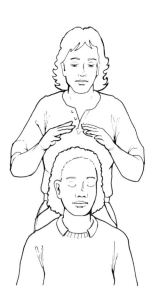

Fig. 42 The Chakra Scan. Starting at the crown chakra.

chakras or in the linking system. A block of stored energy like this is felt as a slight resistance to your own gentle movements.

Make a note of any resistance you sense and where it occurs. This will give you guidance on the possible cause of the condition, as it appears within the etheric body. It will also indicate where healing might be needed at this level.

EXERCISE 80: The Chakra Scan

In this scan, the technique of sensing the etheric energy system becomes your second healing skill.

○ Stand to one side of your patient and hold your hands above the crown chakra. Relax your hands so that the fingers separate naturally (Fig. 42). As in the aura scan, you are not directing healing at this stage but are collecting energetic information about your patient's chakra system.

Make sure that you are as relaxed as possible so that you can focus on what your hands and intuition are telling you.

○ After holding your hands above the crown chakra for a minute or two, move them gently to the brow centre. Your hands are held a few inches from the brow and opposite it at the back of the skull. They do not touch the head. Hold them opposite the brow chakra for a minute or two then move your hands down slowly and gently, without touching the patient's body until they are opposite the front and back of the throat chakra.

○ Continue the scan in this way until you reach the base chakra. You may need to sit comfortably on a chair at the side of your patient. Just make sure your feet are touching the ground at all times.

○ During the chakra scan you may have felt energy leaving your hands or being projected from your patient's chakra system or even nothing at all. Note the different sensations produced by the chakras. This gives you an idea of the balance of the system and where healing might be needed.

With the third scan you move down to the physical level to obtain energetic information about its state of balance and need for healing. This scan should be done with the hands held two or three inches from the body.

EXERCISE 81: The Physical Scan

○ Starting at the head, hold your hands over the skull. Move them slowly and gently down over the back of the skull and down the neck, noting where your patient's body seems to be taking in energy. Move your hands slowly and gently down the back to the base of the spine.

○ This first part of the scan has dealt with the back of the head, neck, vertebral column and central nervous system. Now scan the two sides of the back. Return to the head and move your hands slowly and gently from the forehead, down over the face, throat and front of the body. Scan each side of the trunk, from armpit to pelvis. Again, note where you feel healing is needed by the parts concerned.

○ Now go to the left shoulder. Keep one hand at the shoulder while the leading hand moves down to the elbow. Bring the other hand up to the elbow while the leading hand moves down to the wrist and over the left hand. Still on the left side of the body, hold one hand near the pelvis and move the leading hand down the thigh to the knee. Bring the other hand up to the knee while the leading hand moves down to the ankle and over the left foot.

○ Go to the right side of the body and carry out a scan of the right arm and leg in the same way (Fig. 43).

○ Make a mental note of those parts of the physical body which called for healing.

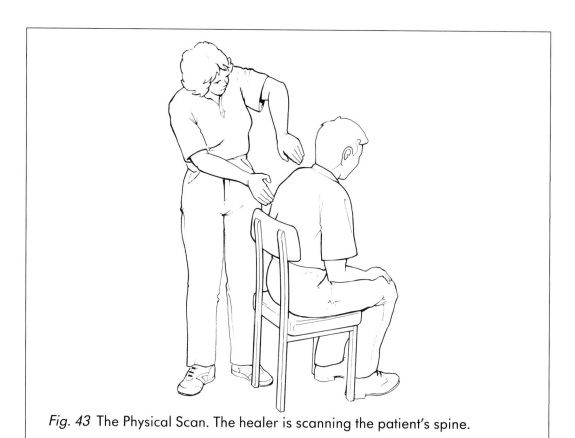

Fig. 43 The Physical Scan. The healer is scanning the patient's spine.

COMPLETING THE TREATMENT

You now have a complete energetic picture of your patient. It is time to use this information to complete the treatment. This is done by returning to where you felt healing was needed as you carried out the three scans.

If you feel impressed to return to any part of the aura, move your hands slowly and gently back there. You may sense energy leaving your hands – a sure sign that you are in the right place. Keep your hands here until you feel that this part of the healing is complete.

Having already noted the state of balance of the patient's chakra system and those chakras where healing was needed, begin to work at this level, keeping the hands a few inches away from the patient's body at all times. Start at the

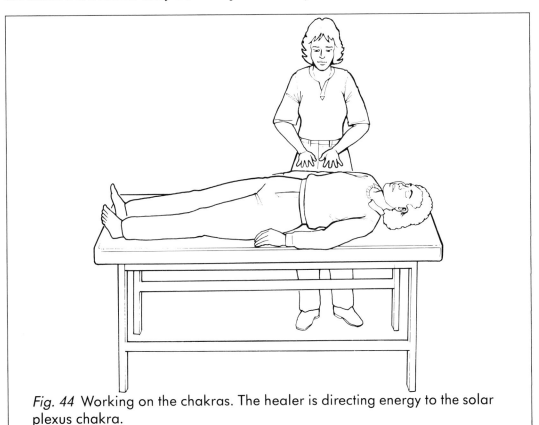

Fig. 44 Working on the chakras. The healer is directing energy to the solar plexus chakra.

base chakra and work your way upwards towards the crown (the direction of the evolutionary force of the chakric energies).

Hold your hands opposite the relevant chakra for as long as it seems to need it. Always move from one chakra to another smoothly and gently and do not make any sudden movements (Fig. 44).

If you wish to balance your patient's chakra system after working on it, carry out Exercise 24: *Balancing The Chakras*, in Chapter 5. If you are unable to pick up any impressions from the chakra scan, carry out the balancing exercise as a matter of course.

Now return to those parts of the physical body which called for healing and keep your hand there for as long as you need to.

If your patient has asked for healing for a specific condition and has no objection to hands-on treatment, it may be appropriate at this point for the patient to feel your hands actually touching the area of the condition, as in, say, an arthritic knee. When the healing is felt as heat, this can be very comforting for the sufferer.

If your patient has not come with any specific condition, you can use the scan method as a way of giving healing and balance to the whole body. Simply carry out the scan, slowly and gently, pausing where you need to, with the intention of channelling healing to the physical body.

It may be helpful to discuss with your patient what you found during the scans, asking them if they can corroborate your findings in any way. Avoid the temptation to 'diagnose'. Rather, encourage *your patient* to talk about her or his condition if you feel this might be helpful.

Like you, your patient may experience healing energies in many ways. They may be felt as heat or cold, movement or vibration. They may be seen as colours, flashes, pictures or other images. They may be sensed as sounds, scents, or feelings. Your patient may feel invigorated, very relaxed, drowsy, light-headed, heavy, or thirsty.

Since it is often necessary, your patient may be conscious of having left her or his body during the healing. If s/he wishes to talk about this experience, show that you accept it and give assurance that such experiences are quite normal and natural.

Be prepared for any observers to have a range of experiences too. They may notice a change in the atmosphere as the healing begins. They may feel a change in temperature or see colours around the patient. I have known friends of patients to fall asleep, feel quite emotional, some even describe their feelings as a sort of religious experience.

I generally feel invigorated during a healing session and this persists until the end of the day. Very often there is a heightening of the senses and an awareness of working at different levels. (I will discuss this aspect in more detail in the next chapter.)

At the end of the session you need to make sure that both you and your patient are back in your bodies. This is the second meaning of 'grounding'. Ask your patient to focus on the feet, wiggle the toes, rub the hands together and breathe deeply. If necessary, you should do the same.

If your patient seems drowsy after a healing session, give them time to return to normal consciousness. Some people need to lie down, so you may need this facility. When you come to know that you will be working with a patient who reacts in this way, bear it in mind when you are organizing your healing day.

Healing opens the energy system so patients should be asked to close up their chakras a little and then to visualize the golden sphere of protection around them, as described in Exercise 30, Chapter 5. This empowers your patients and sends an affirmation to the mind that they are in control of and responsible for their own health. Only when this has been done and you are sure your patients are properly grounded will they be ready to leave and return to everyday activities or drive a car.

Now is the time to accept your fee and to arrange the next appointment if this is necessary.

BREAKING THE LINK

Once your patients have put themselves in their own light of protection, you can recall that your aura now encloses only you. This is the first stage of breaking the temporary link you have made with them. It ensures that you do not transfer the condition of one patient to another, at a subtle level, and that you are free to deal with the next patient. To complete the disconnection, some healers like to wash their hands with water while others visualize their hands being cleansed with light.

Once the patient has left, the healing chair or couch should be cleared as part of the disconnection process and in readiness for the next patient. Visualize silver light cleansing the chair or couch. You have completed your work with your first patient, well done!

CHILDREN AND HEALING

A great many children are natural healers and make excellent channels for the energies if they are allowed to be present when another person or child is receiving healing. Children often show this ability from a young age by wanting to be with the sick or tend sick animals. It is wonderful when parents encourage and support their child healers so that their inborn abilities can develop and be used to help others.

I have found that sick children are very receptive to healing and wholly enjoy a hands-on session. If a small child needs to be held by her or his mother, simply work with the child in this position. If the child frets, you can work in the distant healing mode.

In law, a child is a person under the age of 16, and by law children should first be taken by their parents or guardian to see their doctor if there is a medical condition. This should always be clarified when the appointment is made. If parents do not wish their children to see a doctor first, make sure they sign a statement to this effect. The CHO advises healers to use the following statement:

I have been warned by (name of healer) *that according to law I must consult a doctor concerning the health of my child* (name of child).
Signed (parent or guardian) .... *Date* ....
Signed by witness (signature of person witnessing) ....

Like adults, children can suffer from notifiable or infectious diseases. When this is the case, tell the parents to visit their doctor first and that you will send distant healing until the child is no longer infectious. You would then be happy to see the child.

Children should be treated in the same way as your other patients, with love, care and attention.

REVIEWING THE SESSIONS

It is good policy to review your healing sessions. Were you relaxed and attuned or worried about results? Think about your communication skills. Did you make your patients feel at ease so that they could express their feelings? Did you listen without interrupting? Did you jump to conclusions before waiting to

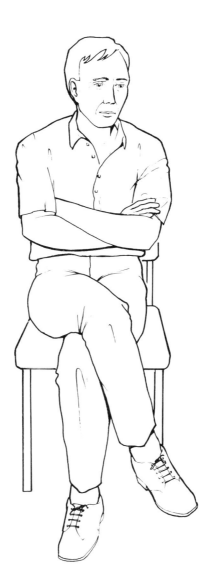

Fig. 45 Defensive body language. The healer is defending his body and covering the solar plexus chakra. The message is: 'I need to defend myself, I'm not confident, neither am I sympathetic to you as a person'.

see what higher forces needed you to do? Did you find yourself making a diagnosis?

Body language is important. Did your body say you were feeling vulnerable or uninterested (Fig. 45)? Did your eyes or face signal disapproval or non-acceptance at any time?

Some patients do not wish to say much while others need to talk before they can accept healing from you. Listening and attention skills are vital to good healing. The skill of demonstrating empathy originates in the heart chakra and is necessary so that you can enter your patient's world and understand what s/he is thinking and feeling. This world should then be left behind once you have disconnected from the patient.

If you find that more and more of your patients seem to need counselling, you should first of all make sure you are realistically aware of the limits of your own counselling skills and stay within these limits. If this aspect of the work appeals to you, it would be a good idea to join a counselling course with a view to upgrading your skills (see Useful Addresses).

Finally, at the end of a day of healing, do not forget to clear yourself and close down using the exercises you have already learned.

You now have enough knowledge and experience of the exercises to begin to work seriously as a responsible healer. But remember that you are just beginning. From now on, every patient who comes to you will bring conditions which will broaden and develop your own way of working. You will be learning from them, as much as they are benefiting from you. It will be a good plan to review your work every six months to see how your development has progressed.

The next task you can enter in your journal is how to integrate your work as a healer with your personal development programme. The next chapter will show you how to take your work a stage further.

13

Healing –
Taking It Further

*T*om sat in the healing chair with a faint smile on his face. He was totally relaxed and at peace. Five minutes earlier he had been looking glum.

'I feel like a hypochondriac,' he had said. 'There's always been something wrong with me.'

There had been a number of unhappy events in Tom's life and he was in the process of coming to terms with them through counselling and healing. One of his permanent conditions was a hiatus hernia. He frequently had mild bouts of asthma too. He described incidents in his life which seemed to rise to the surface as he focused on the area of his hiatus hernia. I was working with the solar plexus chakra, which seemed to 'come alive' as he talked. Healing energy was pouring into this chakra.

Then I became aware of what seemed like two growths on the etheric level, projecting some three or four inches out of Tom's neck. Very gently I took hold of the first 'growth' and pulled it a fraction. Tom's eyes were closed.

'Can you feel that?' I asked.

'Something's pulling in my neck.'

'Is it uncomfortable?'

'No, not at all.'

'There's something sticking out of you on the etheric level which needs to be removed. Tell me if it's uncomfortable or painful,' I said.

I started to pull the etheric protrusion and had drawn out about four inches when I felt a resistance. 'When you can feel me pulling, Tom, I want you to let go, as if you're unclenching your fist.'

Tom 'let go' inside his neck and the rest of the protrusion came out. I felt an unseen hand take it from me and dissolve it. The second protrusion needed a little more work on Tom's part. A particular person, whom he had earlier called to mind, needed to be forgiven and let go of. Did he understand?

Tom nodded and smiled. 'I know what I have to do,' he said.

After a few moments I took hold of the second protrusion and it slid from the base of his throat like a knife coming out of butter.

Tom started with surprise and put his hand over his hiatus hernia. 'Something's happened here. I felt something go!'

Tom's symptoms of burning in the chest cleared up and did not return. He had begun to heal himself.

WORKING WITH THE ETHERIC BODY

Before I worked with Tom, I knew that certain healers worked entirely on the etheric body of their patients. They are able to do this because they are aware of this body through their well-developed high sense perception. It is essential to reach a high degree of awareness of this level before attempting to heal it in this way, and even then it should *only* be used if it is the appropriate treatment for the patient.

In this chapter I will be introducing various ways of working with the etheric body, including common phenomena which you may encounter with patients like Tom.

Once you have mastered all the techniques of *The Healing Session* (Chapter 12), and feel confident about them, the material in this chapter will give you the opportunity to extend your experience. Try the exercises to see if any of the ways of working appeal to you. If they do, you should find that they can be incorporated in your routine quite easily.

Always proceed at the pace which is comfortable for you and consolidate everything that you do, slowly but surely. Your way is right for you, so it is part of your responsibility to yourself to discover the elements of your way. This book is a guide and it may be reassuring for you to find that the ways of working to which you are being drawn are a natural part of your development as a healer. Always remember, however, that the needs of your patient come first. Proper attunement will ensure that your treatment or way of working is guided by your inner links with the patient.

DISTANT HEALING – TAKING IT FURTHER

You learned in Chapter 11 that distant healing is effective over any distance because healing energies originate outside of the space/time dimension of the physical plane. It is also common for healers to work on the astral level during the sleep state. This is why patients frequently report healers appearing in their dreams, talking to them and giving them healing of various kinds. When you consider that all of us leave our bodies during the sleep state, this fact is understandable and not so surprising.

But some healers find they are able to move consciously onto the astral level to carry out distant healing during their waking state. This can happen in two ways when the healer sits for distant healing. They find that either they 'travel' to the person needing help or that person is brought to them in their astral body. Some distant healers like to work this way when there is an emergency call for help or when their healing list is short enough for them to give up the time which is required.

To discover if you can work like this, carry out the following exercise.

EXERCISE 82: Advanced Distant Healing

○ Prepare yourself thoroughly for distant healing as described in Exercise 78 (Chapter 11), and make sure you are properly attuned.

○ Take the first case on your distant healing list and ask to be used as a channel for healing for this person (mention them by name – the vibration of the name makes the linkup).

○ Close your eyes. Even if you do not know the person and have no idea what s/he looks like, sense that the person is there in front of you. Ask how you can be of help.

   If you have been taken to the person, or s/he has been brought to you, you will sense that s/he is in front of you. This becomes easier when you relax and accept that it is possible for this to happen. You will also be able to sense whether the person, child or baby, is lying or sitting in front of you, and where his or her head is, so that you are correctly orientated. As in hands-on healing, use your intuition, inner guidance or inner voice which is directing you, to show you where to put your hands.

Let's take a simple example as explanation. Your help has been asked for a child who has just had an operation on the throat. In this case, you feel drawn to putting your hands over the throat of the child who is in front of you (Fig. 46). If your senses accurately interpret what the child needs, you will feel healing energy leave your hands – or whatever sign tells you that you are working. Keep them there until you feel the healing is complete. You may need to give healing elsewhere so remain aware.

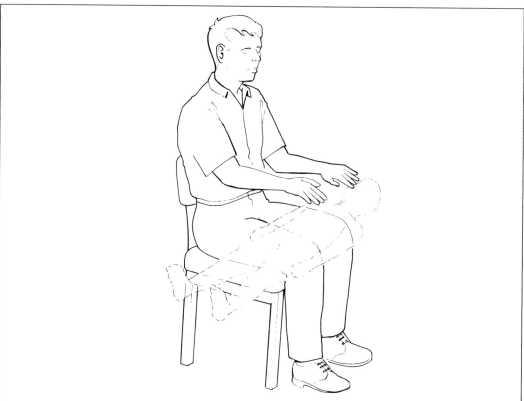

Fig. 46 Advanced distant healing. The healer directs healing to the child's throat as if the child is physically present.

Do not for a moment think that this is all happening in your imagination. A person with high sense perception would be able to 'see' what was going on and confirm that you were working in this way. You are in a sacred space doing sacred work.

○ When you have finished with the first person on your list, thank the person at a soul level and surround him or her with a protective sphere of light. This may be done mentally or by moving your hands to make a sphere around the body (see below).

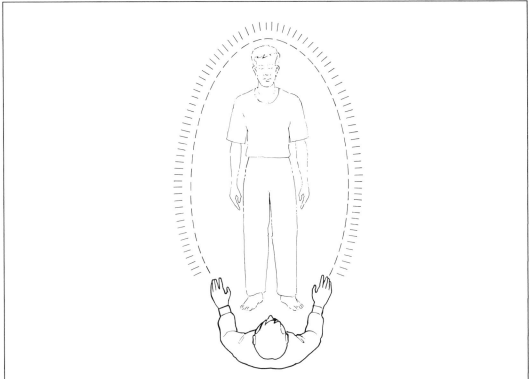

Fig. 47 Distant healing – the Sphere of Protection. The healer directs a sphere of protective light to surround the distant healing patient before closing the session.

○ The distant healing patient then returns to his or her physical body (or the healer does the same).

○ Break the link with the patient by visualizing clearing light washing over your upraised palms. You can now proceed to the next person on the list, if there is one.

I recommend that you start with one patient in this way and build up to six at any one session. It should be remembered that you use up energy through the level of concentration needed to work in this way so it can be tiring. Make a note in your journal of your impressions. If you intend to work like this on a regular basis, keep a record of what happens just as you would with your hands-on patients.

LEVELS OF HEALING

The etheric body is our way into the subtle bodies and their energies and we enter them through the chakras, the 'gateways of light'. The seven major chakras (see Chapter 4), aligned with the spinal cord, represent the human evolutionary journey in terms of our moving through levels of consciousness to our reconnection with the Higher Self or soul. These levels of consciousness are the whole of human experience through which we must travel in order to be totally integrated beings on the physical plane. It is on these levels that we experience problems, deal with issues or don't deal with them, express their energies or do not express them, or store up negative energies as blocks to the flow. So these levels of consciousness are essentially levels of healing (Fig. 48).

WORKING WITH THE CHAKRAS

The chakras link the various bodies or layers of the aura so that they access all emotional, mental and spiritual states of our being. You can see therefore, that being able to work with the chakras is a powerful healing tool which will enhance your ability to help your patients.

Of course, many patients are not interested in their soul's progress, but the cause of their condition is often accessible through the chakras, and this is

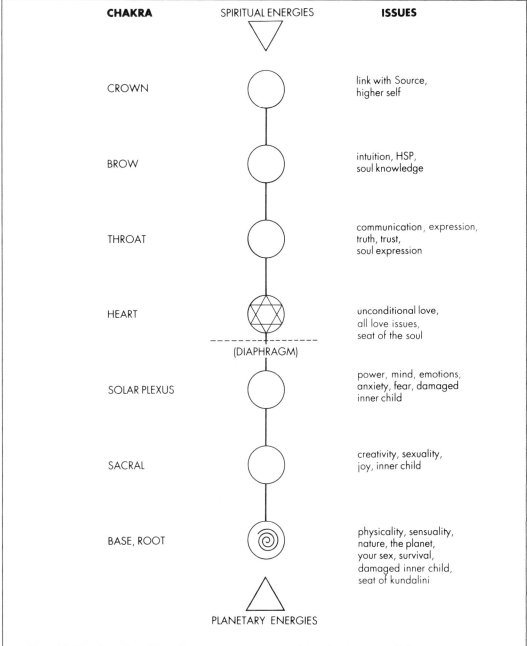

CHARKA   SPIRITUAL ENERGIES   **ISSUES**

CROWN — link with Source, higher self

BROW — intuition, HSP, soul knowledge

THROAT — communication, expression, truth, trust, soul expression

HEART — unconditional love, all love issues, seat of the soul

(DIAPHRAGM)

SOLAR PLEXUS — power, mind, emotions, anxiety, fear, damaged inner child

SACRAL — creativity, sexuality, joy, inner child

BASE, ROOT — physicality, sensuality, nature, the planet, your sex, survival, damaged inner child, seat of kundalini

PLANETARY ENERGIES

Fig. 48 The levels of healing, as represented by the issues of the seven major chakras.

where you can work to help them. For others, healing indirectly shows them where they are on their journey when it points up the issues which they need to address.

The way a person has addressed issues in their life will determine whether s/he has stored energetic material in the chakras, creating a block to energy flow. (A full discussion of energy blocks was given in Chapter 5.) In more advanced work with the chakras you can begin by helping your patient identify any blocks using the following exercise. You will need to work with a partner.

EXERCISE 83: Identifying Energy Blocks in the Chakras

This exercise is similar to Exercise 23, *Sensing Colour in the Chakras, with a Partner* (Chapter 4). The aim is to look for clues to energy blocks as well as to assess the balance of the system. You are going to scan the chakras, starting at the base.

○ Have your partner sit comfortably with the feet flat on the floor and hands resting uncrossed on the thighs.

○ Your partner should then take three full breaths and relax the body.

○ Stand or sit at one side of your partner, with your most sensitive hand opposite the base chakra, a few inches away from it. Put your other hand opposite the throat chakra.

○ Ask your partner to focus on the base chakra and wait until s/he sees a colour on their internal screen. Ask your partner to tell you what colour s/he sees. Is it pale or dark, cloudy or light, blotchy or irregular around the edge and is there a dark patch in the middle?

○ When you have a complete picture of the state of the base chakra, make a mental note of it and move on to the sacral chakra. You may feel an energy block as a slight resistance in the chakras or between them. Make a mental note of this also, to compare with your partner's awareness and what you find out together at the end of the exercise.

○ Ask your partner to clear his or her internal screen and focus on the sacral chakra. Put your most sensitive hand opposite this centre, keeping your other hand opposite the throat chakra to help your partner communicate.

○ When you have completed the scan on all seven chakras, discuss your findings with your partner.

   If you think of a perfectly balanced chakra in terms of the internal screen, the correct colour will be present evenly across the screen. Any change of colour – say, yellow in the base chakra – indicates an imbalance in the system. Any irregularities in the colour indicate small to large energy blocks according to what your partner sees. A dark patch in the middle of the screen is a definite, long-standing block which is having detrimental effects on the person and needs to be addressed as soon as possible.

○ Change roles and let your partner help you identify any energy blocks. Discuss your work together.

○ You could now apply healing by holding your hands over the identified energy blocks, to see if they will take in energy. The healing is complete when all the blocks have been treated in this way.

Some patients will be able to take the work a step further with the next exercise. Here, the chakras are scanned to identify the issue which is the cause of energetic material being stored in the system. This exercise could be carried out at the next session with your patient. However, if your patient feels ready, you could combine it with the previous exercise as one piece of work. Again, you are going to scan the chakras, starting at the base.

EXERCISE 84: Identifying Chakra Issues

○ Have your partner sit comfortably as in the previous exercise.

○ Your partner should take three full breaths and relax the body on the out-breath.

○ Stand or sit at the side of your partner with your most sensitive hand opposite this centre, a few inches away from it. Put your other hand opposite the throat chakra. This will help your partner communicate and express what s/he senses.

○ Ask your partner to focus on her or his base chakra and wait patiently until a symbol, person or event appears on the internal screen.

You may feel energy hitting your hand as your partner focuses and/or gets in touch with an issue. Energy may leave your hand if the chakra is taking in healing. Or the chakra may seem inactive.

○ When something does appear on your partner's internal screen, s/he should tell you what it is and what it means to her or him as it is being seen. Only when your partner has worked as much as s/he wishes to with the image should you move to the sacral chakra. Ask your partner to clear the screen before refocusing.

○ Proceed in the same way with all the seven chakras. Spend a few minutes helping your partner to see if there is a pattern to the images and to work out her or his own interpretation of them. Did there seem to be an issue which needed healing?

Your partner may sense nothing at all, in which case you can talk about the implications of this.

○ Change over and let your partner work with you. Compare final notes together about the exercise. If you have just worked with the previous exercise, how do your findings compare with the identified energy blocks?

When you use this exercise in a healing session, start in the same way, at the base chakra. Once an issue appears on your patient's internal screen, keep your hands at the relevant chakra and help her or him to work with the image while you direct healing to the centre (Fig. 49).

You can help your patients work with an issue by asking them how they relate to the image. Then see if they can discover their own solution to the issue.

Let your hands be alert to the sequence of events which occurs when working with the chakra system in this way. First, energy is released from a chakra when the focus has been made or an issue contacted. Then energy leaves your hand to work on the chakra and facilitate the patient's own efforts.

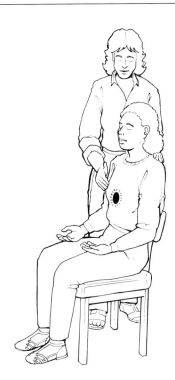

Fig. 49 Working with energy blocks. Here the block is located between the solar plexus and heart chakras. Healing is applied during the session to remove the block, helped by the patient's inner work.

When material is finally released from the chakra, energy is directed again to complete the healing.

It may take more than one session to remove a block, but you will detect a change in the system each time. Always proceed at the pace which is comfortable for the patient.

HEALING GUIDES AND HELPERS

As your high sense perception develops, you will find it invaluable for work on the subtle bodies. The important thing is to remember to work within your capabilities at all times. In this way you will be in control of yourself and your work. This is what your patients need and it is what they should be able to expect.

A great many healers are aware of receiving help from other 'people' who are present on higher frequency vibrations than the physical. You may see them or sense them in some way through high sense perception. Quite often these people seem to be exceptionally qualified and actually carry out the healing task. They are able to be present through the force field created by the healer.

These people are known as 'spirit', 'spirit guides', 'spirit teachers' or 'spirit helpers', according to their role. The word 'spirit' is a useful convention to describe beings on many diverse frequencies who are clearly not in a physical body but who come to take part in the healing work. It should be understood that these beings come out of love alone and their only motive is to help.

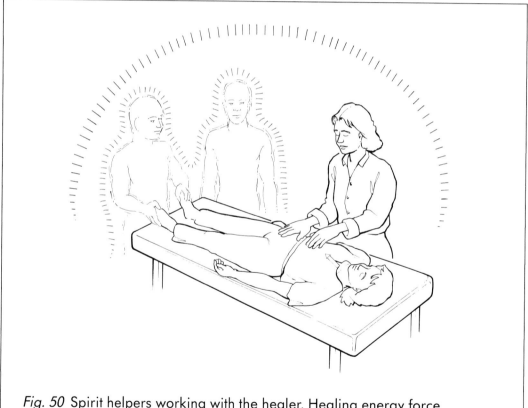

Fig. 50 Spirit helpers working with the healer. Healing energy force field shown.

I feel that most healers are being guided, taught and helped in this way, even if they do not acknowledge it. What could be more natural? The advantage of such a partnership is that you have access at any time to expert help, no matter what condition you have to deal with.

I am often aware of my spirit guides and helpers, there being a great range of them, and it is always a pleasure when someone else is aware of them too. Often, when I am working on certain conditions, I feel other hands moving beneath my own as an 'operation' is carried out with great ease and dexterity. This is frequently confirmed by patients who say they can feel things happening to them in the same part of their body (Fig. 50).

It seems obvious to me that when a surgeon passes over he may well want to go on working. He can do this quite easily in his astral or etheric body and is no longer subject to the restrictions of the physical. I was once made vividly aware of this when working on a patient's bladder with my wife. She could see a spirit surgeon at work and saw exactly what he was doing. Suddenly he turned to her and said with relish, 'It's been a long time since I've done one of these!'

The whole subject of spirit teachers and helpers is vast. You have probably known your healing teacher before and it is very likely that you go for instruction during your sleep state. You may have been together for many lifetimes. Your teacher gathers many other spirit helpers who can work in your aura so that this team of helpers is always there to back you up.

Spirit helpers work at all levels and will help the patient at these levels if required to do so. But this will depend on the quality of your energy field. At the highest levels, they will appear as angelic forms, some quite formless as true beings of light. Now you can understand the need for proper attunement, for the level of your attunement will determine the levels of help which will be available, via you, to your patient.

It should be appreciated by healers, who are aware of what their spirit helpers are saying and doing, that to convey any of this to the patient may not be either helpful or appropriate. Further, it is against the Code of Conduct (mentioned earlier) to give this kind of information to a patient in the form of a 'clairvoyant reading' during the actual healing session. This is to prevent what may be false information being given to a trusting patient under the guise of 'higher teachings'. Use your common sense with all inner guidance and use your discretion as to how you convey this to others, if at all. Self deception destroys the work. Your throat chakra will always advise you to be truthful.

This aspect of spiritual healing is not there to mystify or impress, but to demonstrate the depth of love which surrounds us, even though we are rarely aware of it or in tune with it.

I do not include exercises to help your spirit teachers and helpers to 'come through'. Simply relax and work normally, allowing your awareness to develop naturally. It is far more important to get on with the healing than wonder who might be looking over your shoulder.

WORKING WITH NEGATIVE ETHERIC MATERIAL

Working with your hand an inch or two from your patient's body gives you much more scope for sensing the energy patterns of the physical and etheric bodies. Many physical conditions are actually being held in place by an energetic etheric counterpart, either close to the problem or in other parts of the body. This is because the physical body is directly affected by what is going on in the etheric.

Energetic material being stored in the etheric body sets up energy blocks which act on the physical body. Very often the body signals this disturbance through a specific condition, as in Tom's case.

Healers with well-developed high sense perception are able to look into the etheric body and see the forms taken by negative energies which are being stored there, or they can sense them in other ways. Some healers with these abilities know how to extract these forms in order to bring balance back to the etheric body and to help restore the health of the physical. The healer and writer Betty Shine, for example, is able to work in this way.

I am sharing my own experience with you, and you can use this as a reference point. I am not always visually aware of the etheric body, rather I tend to sense it. I was therefore very surprised the first time I became aware of negative etheric material actually protruding from a patient's body when it hadn't been there earlier on in the healing session.

'Rods' were sticking out of the patient's back some six inches. I assumed this was not a good way to be and that they needed to be removed. I felt I could remove them if I was careful. My first precaution was to see if my patient was also aware of them. I tweaked them gently, one by one. Yes, she could feel them. (If the patient is not aware of such things I always wait until the time comes when they are aware in some way.) I pulled the rods out, just as I described with Tom, very slowly and gently, pausing where there was resistance until the resistance was removed by the patient's inner work (Fig. 51).

Etheric material which needs to be removed can be experienced in many ways – as a liquid, as lumps, as a mass within the etheric body, as threads, as

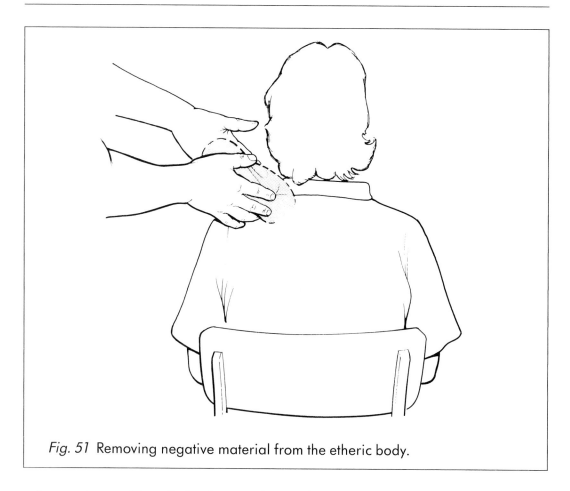

Fig. 51 Removing negative material from the etheric body.

spines, and so on. They all give the same impression, which can sometimes be quite unpleasant, that they should not be there.

I do not look for this kind of material, but I find that my attention is drawn to it during certain healing sessions. On these occasions I am very aware of my spirit helpers. As I extract the material, it is dissolved by them. It is important to know what is happening at this stage – you cannot just throw the material away and hope it will disappear. It is an energy and must be dealt with responsibly.

A good rule of thumb in healing is to treat the whole being of your patient with respect. The physical body, the subtle bodies and aura are part of their sacred space. This attitude will ensure that you honour them and the work.

WORKING WITH ANIMALS, PLANTS AND THE PLANET

Another way of extending your healing practice is to give help to the other kingdoms – animal, vegetable and mineral. The work of those who have contacted these kingdoms, such as Dorothy Maclean, has shown us that they, too, have a need for healing (see Further Reading). We have brought about tremendous imbalances through our interaction with these kingdoms and it is up to us to restore health and harmony by healing what has been damaged. If you are drawn to this work there are subtle forces waiting to assist you.

ANIMALS

Before treating an animal, you should make sure that it has been examined by a veterinary surgeon. If not, you should advise the owner to do this. It is important to remember that, in law, the veterinary surgeon remains in charge of the case and that neither instructions nor medicines should be countermanded by a healer.

However, under the Veterinary Surgeons Act, it is permissible for healers to give healing in an emergency for the purpose of saving life or to relieve pain. Animal owners should be assured that spiritual healing is a complementary therapy and can in no way interfere with other therapeutic practice. On the contrary, my experience has shown that it can positively enhance the work of other therapies.

When you find animals being brought to you, it may be a sign that this will be part of your practice. Most animals respond very satisfactorily to healing. They slip from physical consciousness to the etheric and astral levels quite normally and this makes it easy to work with them. I have found that healing normally pacifies an animal and frequently sends them to sleep – the sign that they have left their physical body. Animals like hands-on healing, but they respond equally well to distant healing.

Sometimes a nervous animal is best left with its owner until it calms down. In this case, start with distant healing until the animal is pacified. Animals suffering from mental, emotional or physical trauma need to be treated with kindness, care and gentleness. If you can put your hand anywhere on the animal's body, the energies will flow to where they are required. If not, hold your hands near the animal or do your whole treatment on a distant healing basis.

Animals have a chakra system which may be sensed in their etheric bodies, but it is not necessary to try to locate their chakras. Simply work intuitively, putting your hands where they want to go and where the body is asking for healing.

Do not work with animals you *fear*. Address your fear or aversion first (yes, even snakes and other reptiles sometimes need healing!) so that you are confident and positive in your approach to them. The only limits to animal healing are those which we impose ourselves.

Keep records of all your sessions with animals just as you would with your human patients.

PLANTS

As you may have found in Exercise 75: *Sensing the Energy Field of a Plant* (Chapter 11), plants respond to healing very quickly. This is frequently the case with house plants where owners fail to maintain the balance of conditions necessary for the plant's good health.

Outside, or in your own garden, you will discover individual plants or whole areas of plants which need your help. As you travel about, you will find many opportunities to work with the plant kingdom, and this includes trees. The landscape is continually being devastated by road-building, development, housing, even forestry and farming. If you visit these areas your hands will soon tell you what is needed.

If you want to help plants, start with the ones nearest to you. You can monitor these and see how your healing is helping them. Most plants like to be touched. Apart from trees and large shrubs, this has to be quite gentle. But healing can be done by holding the hands a few inches from the plants or even at a distance. Plants that have to be pruned or damaged in some way appreciate your concern when it means you send them healing.

THE PLANET

You live on part of the planet. Unless you are very fortunate, it is certain that not far from you an area of the planet needs help. The mineral kingdom has an evolutionary path just like we do and there is great work to be done to try to align human demands with the needs of the landscape, the soil, metals, gems, rocks and stones.

If you have a deep feeling for the environment, you will find it enlightening to find out about the wisdom of aboriginal cultures, such as the American, Australian and Polynesian, with their positive attitudes and teachings about the ground beneath your feet. These cultures have much to offer in the field of planetary healing.

Best of all, start with your own intuitive guidance on what to do about a ravaged landscape in terms of healing. You may be pleasantly surprised to find later that your practice was close to that of healers living far from you in other countries. As always, your hands will know what to do and your heart will be a better guide than your mind.

Don't forget that working with the planet is a spiritual exercise. All the steps you take to attune before and to close down after are necessary.

Patients like Tom may be extending the scope of your work. A traumatized animal or damaged meadow may be calling to you. Whatever the case, part of the great adventure and challenge of healing is to go with what is presented to you. I believe that whatever condition has come your way, it has arrived at your door because you are the right person to do the job. Like attracts like and you will attract what you need to work with. Put your trust in the highest, ask to be a channel for the best and expect the best.

It is not up to the healer to impose a technique on patients, rather to facilitate their getting in touch with what *they* need.

Over the years, patients have shown me how they choose to use the healing energies directed to them to show themselves what the true nature of their energy imbalance is. Going with what the patient presents has opened up whole new areas of healing to me.

Healers have this confidence when they feel the energies of love flowing through them. And love will always take your healing that one step further.

14

Birth, Reincarnation and The Inner Child

L esley found herself in a dark cave lit by a strange green light. The walls of the cave seemed to be covered with various kinds of moss which dripped with moisture. She looked about the cave and did not like the feeling of claustrophobic dampness which was bearing down on her.

She fidgeted in her seat and swallowed hard. 'I want to get out of here, I don't like it.'

Lesley's sacral chakra was at last beginning to take in energy, at the same time her solar plexus needed calming. A feeling of frustration was building up inside her, making her very uncomfortable.

'I want to move my legs, but I can't. Help me, please!'

I knew that she would not let herself leave 'the cave' until this part of the healing was complete, but I encouraged her to look for a way out. The level of energy pouring into her sacral chakra began to drop. At last Lesley saw some light and went towards it. She had to climb up rocks to get to the light but she finally made her way out and found herself in a clearing at the edge of a forest.

She sighed with relief. 'I don't want to go back there again.'

I asked her to look round and find a place in the clearing where she could rest. In a few moments she went deeper into her memory.

Suddenly she gasped, 'That cave was inside my mother! I was being born, but I couldn't get out.' She shuddered. 'The feeling of not being able to escape was terrible.'

She had shown herself that she needed to heal the memory and that it was possible to go back and do this, for the memory was stored energy she no longer needed. Reluctantly, Lesley agreed. She let herself enter the cave once more. This time it was more open and with a higher ceiling. It glowed with a mysterious but welcoming light.

Her solar plexus chakra had now calmed down completely.

'Do you feel frightened or trapped?' I asked.

'No, I can go where I like.'

She saw what she called 'little treasures' and decided to take some with her as she made her way out of the cave without difficulty. At this point her sacral chakra stopped absorbing energy.

This part of the healing helped Lesley to come to terms with the birth of her own son, a memory she had repressed because of its power to evoke her own traumatic birth.

In a later session, Lesley recalled that her mother had wanted a boy. She grew up not liking herself, especially her own femininity. Her self-disgust was compounded in later life with the complicated birth of her son. By then she had a block in the sacral chakra which could well have exacerbated her own difficulty in giving birth.

Healing has a role to play at all stages of a child's life, from the moment of conception, for healing energy is beneficial for mother, foetus and growing baby. I am always amused when a healing session like Lesley's takes a patient back to her own birth because, in law, spiritual healers are not allowed to attend women in childbirth! But this aspect of childhood may be one which you will be asked to work with – the trauma of childbirth. When this happens, simply apply healing in the normal way and allow your patients to guide you to where *they* need help. As long as you are properly attuned you need have no fear of not knowing what to do.

THE MEANING OF BIRTH

Through working with patients who have presented many conditions linked to conception, pregnancy and birth, I have built up a picture of how and why the individual soul enters the Earth plane.

The soul comes here either to experience, to learn or to express, or a combination of these needs. They may also include the balancing factor of karma (the law of cause and effect). As I have already mentioned, this comes into operation when the soul decides to address imbalances created in past lives. Karmic imbalance can involve other souls or other experiences where learning or expression was not properly achieved.

The soul's needs therefore have a direct influence on the choices to be made about the incarnation. When we decide to come here, we choose our mother and father, the time and place of birth, our name (which carries a vibration influencing our life path and health), and the spiritual environment we will probably grow up in. We will also have decided our own health pattern and whether our role will be to teach or help others if this is what we need to do. Sometimes our role is to provide opportunities for others to learn.

The soul's incarnation choices will in turn affect the creation of the personality (ego) and its pattern of conditioning. This is the aspect of Self through which the soul will experience life and express itself. The effects of the conditioning factors and the soul forces on the growing personality will be discussed later in the chapter.

THE TIMING OF INCARNATION

A number of souls are in touch with the growing embryo, exploring the possibility of incarnation. One will choose to unite with the baby around the time of birth because the conditions seem compatible with this soul's needs. Since most souls decline to experience the trauma of birth, the linkup usually takes place a few moments after. However, some souls link with the baby before, during, or some hours after the birth, according to the circumstances they wish to experience.

The incarnating soul contains the records of all its experiences. Once it incarnates, emanations from this energy pattern rapidly permeate every cell of the body. In this way, the little person begins the task of expressing the soul on the Earth plane. This task may be amplified or thwarted by the problems of balancing it with aspects of personality which have been inherited through genetics and/or conditioning.

It is rare that parents are aware of or understand the needs of the incarnating soul. In 1991, an initiative was formed by cardiac surgeon Michel Bercot and his wife Anne to encourage this awareness and understanding. The Institute of Luminaissance was launched in France to train parents and health professionals in 'the art of welcoming the newly incarnating soul and in facilitating the spiritual purpose of the new-born'.

Naturally, survival is seen by parents as paramount, but my work has shown me that some souls wish to spend only a short time on Earth, and this time may be very brief. The soul is very often prevented from leaving when it wishes through the intervention of well-meaning medical science and the desires of others. If the soul does leave, the baby can only be kept 'alive' through the use of machines or transplants. If the soul has left its body, the baby or child will die no matter what intervention takes place.

Once parents and carers are taught how to communicate with the souls which they have attracted to them, much distress will be avoided on both sides. People will then be able to realize that the relationship with their child does not need to end at death. They simply enter into a new relationship with their child.

LOSING CONTACT WITH THE SOURCE

Birth is traumatic for the physical consciousness which has been developing since conception, because the baby has come from a place of darkness, warmth and comfort, inside its mother, to almost the opposite. The darkness of the womb is indeed the preparatory state for entry into the physical world, contrasting with the place of light from which the soul is coming.

The baby is limited in what it can physically do and will have to endure many years of growth before becoming an independent person in its own right. During this time it depends on others for nourishment, love and care.

The baby tries to accommodate its new experiences by spending much of the time sleeping. This allows it to move its consciousness onto other levels and stay in contact with the Source. But the needs of the growing body, for exercise and acclimatization to Earthly life, mean that the long periods of sleep begin to diminish. By about the age of three, the baby's strong links with the Source have become weakened.

Sensations continue to crowd in to be processed by the brain, and these demands gradually create the illusion of a separate self. The child now becomes more and more aware of its own personality, and the personalities of those around it, as it enters into the experiences of life. For many years it will be strongly influenced by all that happens physically, emotionally, mentally and spiritually.

Then around teenage a re-awakening to inner realities takes place through many different experiences. These may be mystical or religious, sudden overwhelming feelings, deep love for another person. Even the trauma of accident or loss can re-open areas of spiritual consciousness which temporarily had been closed down.

But whether a person responds to the re-awakening or is even aware of it depends on their conditioning and how enclosed in the personality they have become through painful experience. It could be many years before they feel the promptings of the soul.

Once there is an awareness of deep needs, spiritual healing can play an important role in helping people address them. You are responding to inner needs through your interest in healing. With the help of the following exercises, let's look at the long and winding road which your soul journey has followed from the time of your entry to the planet. Don't forget to record all your findings in your journal.

EXERCISE 85: Happy Birthday to You!

Do you know exactly when and where you were born?

○ Find out what you can about your own birth. Make notes about your parents and where they were living at the time. What were the conditions around you then? What was the weather like? Add the astrological details if this interests you.

○ Now see if these factors make a pattern which shows you how they have determined aspects of your personality.

This exercise involves much gathering of facts. The next exercise asks you to think some more about the implications of these facts.

EXERCISE 86: Looking at Birth Choices

○ Try to get in touch with why you chose your particular parents, that particular location, that particular time (which means that you are on the planet *now*).

○ Why do you think you are male or female at this time?

If you find any of these things disturbing, you have probably had some difficult lessons to learn through them or you may need to do some work to identify the lessons.

EXERCISE 87: Looking at the Family

○ What family network is there – brothers, sisters, etc?

○ Where is your place in it and how has the network affected you?

○ How do you think you compare in soul development with the rest of the family?

○ Who do you feel close to and why? Record your answers in your journal.

Your answers to the questions in the last two exercises will tell you a lot about yourself. You are beginning to see a pattern emerge which shows you in which ways your family has played an important role in your soul journey.

All the factors you have discovered in the last three exercises have equipped you for your soul experiences. They provide you with ways of expressing and with ways of learning. Let's look at some of the learning.

EXERCISE 88: The Teenage Years

○ Think back to your teenage years. You may even need to go back to 11 or 12.

○ What events can you recall taking place which, with hindsight, you can see were turning (or trying to turn) your attention to spiritual realities and ideals?

○ What happened as a result? Are they part of your life now?

○ How do you think you have evolved as a person since then? Record your answers in your journal.

EXERCISE 89: The Lessons of Life

○ With the understanding you have acquired from working with the book so far, are you able to rethink what might have seemed to be the 'negative' experiences in your life? Perhaps you have reached a stage in your life where you can identify some of the lessons you have learned. Give yourself a hug for this recognition, especially the painful ones. If you recognize that you have indeed learned these lessons, tell yourself that you do not need to repeat them, and give yourself another hug!

Have you noticed how most of your life experiences have emphasized your separateness rather than your *uniqueness*? Your life of apparent separation has been a great challenge. Perhaps the greatest challenge has been how to find your way back to the Source and oneness. Your response to the next exercise will show you how close you are to becoming aware of a greater sense of reality.

EXERCISE 90: A Greater Sense of Reality

○ See if you can recall any moments when you were aware of a greater reality beyond yourself.

○ What gave you this impression?

○ Make notes about this in your journal.

○ Have there been moments of feeling at one with another person, animal, plant or place?

○ Have there been moments of feeling at one with all things? Try to describe, illustrate or express this experience of oneness in some way.

REINCARNATION – AND REGRESSION BEYOND BIRTH

Many healers have found that some patients seem to need to regress beyond birth, and being carried in their mother's womb, to recall the events of another life altogether. Healer and writer Diana Cooper, for example, has found that many of her patients need to contact other lifetimes to understand their current health condition. In these lives they discover the original cause of a problem which, because it was never healed, keeps appearing in different guises as the signal for attention.

Awareness of past lives is such a common occurrence worldwide that the subject is now very well documented. A report published in India in 1990 by Dr Satwant Pasricha of the National Institute of Mental Health and Neurosciences in Bangalore, detailed 250 cases of reincarnation. Over 25 per cent of the subjects exhibited physical marks, phobias or conditions which could be related to their previous lives.

Dr Pasricha's work complements the accounts of people born with brand marks on their bodies and who can recall past lives as Cathars in Southern France. (Members of this Christian Sect, of 12th and 13th century Provence, were persecuted by the Catholic authorities for their heretical belief that goodness could be found in the spiritual world alone.)

Rabbi Yonasson Gershom's recent book *Beyond the Ashes* (1992), describes the cases of 78 people from many countries who can recall past lives in the Holocaust. Interestingly, 55 of these are not Jewish in this life. In most of the cases, healing was an important outcome of the past life recall (see Further Reading).

I do not encourage any patient to regress to a past life, but if during the healing session this is what happens I will go with it, confident that the patient has the key to his or her own condition. If this happens to you as a healer, I recommend that you carry out your healing in the normal way. Healing energy will still be processed in the way that is best for your patient and this will be ensured by your maintaining a relaxed, open and confident attitude during the course of your work.

But I am sure the experience will encourage you to address the possibility of reincarnation. Simply stay with the policy advocated in this book, which is to build up your own data base, try to keep an open mind, and trust your inner guidance.

Working with patients has convinced me that it is highly unlikely that a soul could experience all that it wishes to experience, learn all that it can learn and express all that it needs to express in the course of one lifetime. Secondly, where the law of cause and effect (karma) means that many of us leave the earth plane with an imbalance of experience to redress, reincarnation gives us the chance to do this.

If reincarnation is a fact, then karmic energies will be discovered in a patient's chakric system and will show up in the aura. This I have found to be the case.

I sometimes look at a patient with awe when I think of the total cosmic journey this soul has already made. Reincarnation puts the whole panorama of human life into a healing perspective. It makes sense of what seems so often to be without purpose, it gives meaning to countless lives of suffering and it promises justice where injustice seems to have gained the upper hand.

INFLUENCES ON CHILD DEVELOPMENT

What stands out in recent reincarnation studies is the number of children who seem able to describe their last life or past lives quite lucidly and who have no problem with the idea of having lived before. Perhaps their ability to accept the apparent fact of reincarnation will help them cope with the problems that life will bring.

Our development as children depends on many factors and influences, which, as we discussed earlier, actually originated at the soul level. But, once we arrive here, they quickly become the facts of life with which the personality must come to terms.

The personality is the embodiment of the soul's choices, which have determined the influence of genetics, family structure, friends, diet, education, planetary forces, environment, health or ill health, and all the conditioning that these factors will bring about.

The personality will also be subject to changes in the environment and world happenings. It will be affected by the soul's ability to adjust to the physical level and later the pressure exerted from this aspect of Self to carry out the soul's mission. Finally it will be influenced by the forces of karma (Fig. 52).

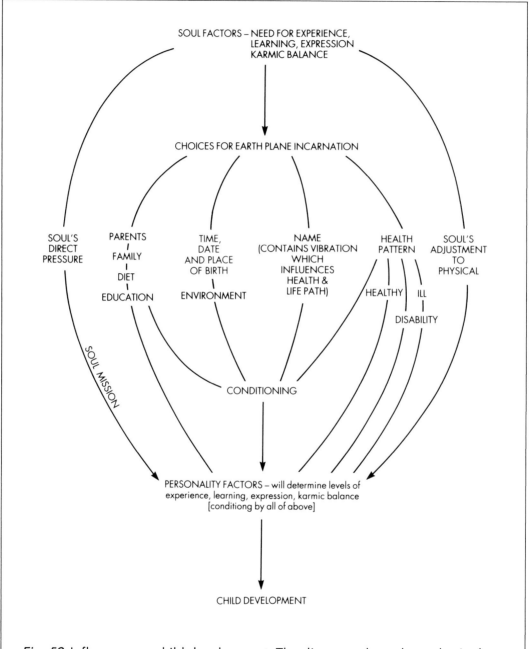

Fig. 52 Influences on child development. The diagram shows how physical influences originate at a soul level.

Since all these factors and influences have a bearing on health it follows that all healing depends on the soul's reasons for coming to Earth.

REVIEWING PAST INFLUENCES

The following exercise helps you to review some of the influences that went to make you the person you think you are today. It should be carried out with a partner.

EXERCISE 91: Looking at Childhood Influences

○ Spend a minimum of 15 minutes talking together about your childhood, focusing on your parents, family, where you were born and when.

○ Then look at the environment you grew up in, your schooling, your friends and all those who had an influence on you. Try not to focus too much on negative influences.

○ Make notes on what you recalled about your childhood that seems particularly significant. Were there any influences which may have begun the quest which led you to work with this book? You are getting back in touch with yourself as a child.

THE INNER CHILD AND THE WOUNDED CHILD

In a healthy, integrated human being there is an aspect of the Higher Self present in the sacral chakra. This is the inner child or soul child. This soul aspect cannot be damaged or harmed in any way. The wisdom of the inner child links us with our creativity and joy and puts the fun into life through play and spontaneity. This aspect of the Self monitors the growth of the personality from childhood to adulthood and holds the key to healing when this growth is inadequate, when it has been interfered with or arrested for some reason.

There is also a child aspect of *personality* within each human being. At the moment when the soul enters the baby, or physical body, these two child aspects – soul and personality – are in perfect alignment. But most of us take on personality factors which break down this alignment.

We all have specific growth needs in terms of love, approval, affection and respect. Most parents, no matter how loving they may be, are unable to satisfy all our needs. Some children have no-one to love them. Others find the love that may be given is undermined by parental behaviour such as violence, abuse, instability, unreliability, absence, and so on.

The most common pattern for many of us, therefore, is one of unfulfilled childhood needs. Practice has shown me that, for many patients, this is compounded by emotional, mental and spiritual trauma.

The moment when the foetus, or baby or small child is first hurt in any way, the alignment with the soul child is broken. This is the point when it becomes what is known as the 'wounded child'. From then on, all further hurts and traumas will increase the ego's sense of separation and loss. Certain key incidents occur which reinforce the wounded child's damaged concepts of herself/himself. These are also known to the inner or soul child.

We cannot stop growing chronologically, but growth on other levels becomes interrupted. Even the growth and development of the physical body can be adversely affected by the knock-on effects of the energy blocks in the chakras. Thus many people find they have an adult body but they do not always feel 'grown up' or behave in a mature way. This is because the wounded child within them is filled with fears, anxieties, anger, frustration and many unfulfilled needs.

So whenever we are in a situation linked to love or emotion, or when someone else's behaviour triggers unconscious memories of past hurts, our wounded child takes the stage and dictates our responses, attitudes and how we feel – the adult behaves like a wounded child.

This also means that we see the world and other people through a veil of pain and confusion and cannot possibly see them as they really are. Unless the wounds of the damaged ego are healed and its demands for emotional growth are met, we may find that this aspect of personality tends to dominate and wreak havoc in our lives.

The next exercise extends the previous one to look at childhood influences which may have caused you pain, perhaps even having a negative effect on your personal growth. Again, it is best carried out with a partner, though it could be attempted as a solo exercise.

EXERCISE 92: Looking at Childhood Hurts

○ Spend a minimum of 15 minutes talking together about painful memories from childhood. Focus on just one or two incidents at first.

○ Try also to be interested, sympathetic listeners. The person talking must feel safe and accepted.

○ As you talk together, other memories may be awakened which you had forgotten about. Try to allow them to come to the surface. Let the conversation flow back and forth until you have both said as much as you want to.

Did you notice anything about your body which changed as the conversation progressed? Were you defensive, wanting to change the subject? Did heartbeat or breathing change? Did you feel queasy in the solar plexus area or pain in the centre of the chest or throat? Talk about these changes together.

Make notes on what you discovered about yourself. This exercise can stand on its own as a way of helping you connect with childhood pain. Even better is to follow it after an hour or two with the next exercise.

WORKING WITH THE WOUNDED CHILD

Through the work of therapists like John Bradshaw, healing the wounded child has come to be highly valued and understood as a powerful therapy in the field of recovery and dysfunctional families (see Further Reading). It is widely known as 'inner' child work, referring to the child aspect of the *ego*. As I have explained, the soul child and personality, or ego, child are two different 'inner' children. The soul child cannot be damaged, conditioned or traumatized, whereas the personality child usually suffers at least two of these effects.

If a healer is asked to work with the patient's inner problems and conflicts, the chakras hold the key to blocked and stored energies so that part of the healing focus will be here. Once energies are directed to this level, either one or both of the inner children may surface, bringing valuable information about crucial incidents and feelings from the past which need healing.

The wounded child appears in one of the lower three chakras. When survival has been threatened, or when there has been physical cruelty or abuse, the wounded child may be found in the base chakra. When fear or anxiety are prominent, or when mental cruelty has been endured, the solar plexus chakra tends to be the place of the wounded child.

In spiritual healing, either the wounded child or inner child or both will present themselves. To the patient they may seem the same and it is not necessary to point out the differences in the early stages of the work. But if the patient wishes to identify them they will recognize the inner soul child as undamaged, free and full of fun. Either child is capable of guiding the healing process, the wisdom of the inner child being especially reliable.

The healer's role is to help the patient get in touch with their wounded and inner child so that the one can show what is damaged, and how it happened, and the other can provide inspirational guidance about the best way to conduct the healing. I include an excerpt from one of Harry's healing sessions to illustrate how this may be done.

'I've often wondered if it started when I was a little boy. What do you think?' Harry asked.

'Is there something that makes you feel this?'

Harry's brow furrowed. He looked out of the window as he put his hand to his mouth and swallowed.

Harry thought there was little point in looking back at childhood from his age of 62, but he seemed to need confirmation that it might help him with his 'groundless fears'. We talked together for some 10 minutes and gradually the conversation opened up Harry's memory.

He found it difficult to hold back the tears as he recalled how his parents could never stop rowing and how their arguments often ended in things being broken. As a little boy he was frightened over and over again. He had buried these memories, yet even now feared the sound of raised voices and found it difficult to make his point in any discussion.

During the healing session, later on, Harry was helped to address the issue which had come up. He had to realize that this had happened because he was ready and able to let go of it. It was an old energy which he no longer needed to store.

First, Harry got in touch with the pain of the issue, saw himself as a little boy and located the pain in the solar plexus chakra. There was also secondary pain in the heart chakra, indicating how the arguments had undermined his love for his parents.

> *'Little Harry' appeared on his inner screen and demanded lots of love and reassurance. He also wanted to speak to his parents and tell them how he had felt when they quarrelled so violently. Harry was amazed to watch his parents appear on his inner screen and to find it so easy for forgiveness and reconciliation to take place. When his parents left the scene, little Harry still needed to be picked up and cuddled and reassured that he was wanted in Harry's adult life.*
>
> *The session proved to be the first of a successful series of healings in which Harry worked with his inner child to bring about emotional wholeness.*

The following exercise allows you to heal a childhood hurt with which you made contact in Exercise 92. It should be carried out with a partner. Alternatively, make a tape allowing for pauses in the appropriate places.

EXERCISE 93: Healing a Childhood Hurt

This should be preceded by an activity or exercise like the previous one which has helped you to get in touch with a childhood issue. This acts as a signal to your inner child that it is safe to present the issue and that you wish to address it. Each partner should read the exercise to the other or you could use the tape together.

○ Light a candle between you and dedicate the light to, say, the healing of all wounded children. Now visualize the light of unconditional love linking your heart chakras and a beam of light linking you to the Source, with a third beam linking your partner to the Source, forming the Healing Triangle. Read out the rest of the exercise to your partner, allowing time for the inner work to be done. This requires you to be alert and sensitive to their needs.

○ Identify the issue which came up in the previous exercise. See yourself at the age when the issue occurred. Let the issue unfold to your inner vision rather than relying on memory. Locate where you feel the issue – somewhere in your body or in a chakra – and let that be your place of focus.

○ Ask the child that you see what s/he needs you to do. Carry out what your child says. If you get no response, do what you feel a child hurting like this would need. This is your act of self-healing.

○ The issue has come up because you are ready and able to let go of it. Now see it surrounded by a ball of light. Take hold of the ball of light, with the issue inside, and let go of it gently. Tell yourself that you no longer need this old energy.

○ There is now a space in you where the old energy used to be. Breathe in love to fill this space. Breathe in peace to fill this space.

○ Take the hand of your inner child and send her or him new, positive messages saying how you feel about her or him. Tell your child how much you love her or him.

○ Still holding the hand of your inner child, go for a walk together. See what your child wishes to show you. When you are both ready, come back in your own time.

○ Make sure that your partner is properly grounded after completing the exercise.

○ If you wish to use this exercise as part of your own self-healing programme, simply follow the procedure as outlined above.

THE PLAYFUL SOUL AND THE WOUNDED PERSONALITY

Working as a spiritual healer with a patient's inner child is specialist work which demands experience, development and a great deal of confidence in your inner guidance. As with all aspects of healing, do not attempt to work in this way until you know what you are doing or there is someone who can supervise you. Having said this, you may be presented with a case where, because you recognize and understand the need, you can offer healing to the patient's wounded child.

I have found that working with the inner child is one of the most effective means to bring about personal integration. If the personality has become damaged because of what happened during the childhood years, the damage creates a barrier to the soul's full expression. So healing works with both of the damaged patient's inner 'children'.

People need to reaffirm their link with their own joy, spontaneity, creativity and sense of fun. By working with either the playful soul, or the wounded personality, spiritual healing releases the 'inner child' to show the adult the way to grow to wholeness and happiness.

When this happens, the alignment that was present at birth is restored and we can safely be 'as little children'.

15

Journey into Light

C laire looked down at the scene below her. People were frantically busying themselves around what looked like her body. She could see that the 'other' Claire lying on the operating table was quite peaceful, but the people around her seemed worried and agitated. 'I wish they would just leave me alone,' she thought. 'I'm quite happy where I am.'

The next moment she found herself travelling at great speed through a tunnel. Light was coming into view at the end of it. She was moving into the light, filled with a profound sense of peace and joy. She could not see them but she was aware that two beings of light were by her side. She was floating now, rather than walking, through a beautiful garden where she could see her father tending some flowers. Her father had died some years before, she recalled. She must be in heaven.

Her father was overjoyed to see her and greeted her with a hug. 'It's wonderful here, Claire, you'll love it, but it's not your time yet – you'll have to go back soon.'

They talked together as they strolled arm in arm. Her father explained that she still had things to do in her Earthly life, she still had a role to play in the lives of her husband and children. Claire felt a pang of sadness at the thought of leaving her father again.

But he reassured her. As he looked into her eyes he said, 'I'll be around, don't you worry. Look out for me. Look at the flowers. Everything will be fine, you'll see.'

One more hug and she was retracing her steps back through the garden, past the trees, admiring a bush which had just come into blossom . . .

'Claire! Can you hear me? Blink if you can hear me.'

She opened her eyes. Many pairs of anxious eyes were looking down at her. She was back. They seemed relieved. She felt angry as intense pain surged through her body. But this could not blot out the reality of her experience. And as the years went by it remained fresh and vivid in her memory.

THE NEAR-DEATH EXPERIENCE

Claire had had a near-death experience (NDE). It changed her previous fear of death to an open and ready acceptance of it, whenever it should actually occur. Every day was a gift in which she could now see a spiritual purpose.

The phenomenon of the near-death experience comes about through the resuscitation of people who have begun the process of dying. They have returned to their physical body and been able to report an experience (the NDE) which is now corroborated by world-wide research across many cultures and religions. The near-death experience has always occurred, but it has only recently become well-reported due to the modern ability to resuscitate people in a clinical setting.

A leading American researcher, Dr Melvin Morse, of Washington University, identifies aspects common to most NDEs. These include a sense of peace, an out-of-body experience, the sensation of travelling through a tunnel, encountering beings of light, a reluctance to return, a review of one's life and a personality transformation brought about by the event. Dr Morse considers that the near-death experience supports the findings of modern physics that we are 'beings of light' (see Further Reading).

Research, such as that being carried out by Dr Morse, is a valuable scientific endorsement of the experiences of healers about the process of dying. Before NDE research, healers would comfort the bereaved and the terminally ill with the benefit of their own knowledge. Today we are in a position where we can quote the near-death experience as further evidence that dying is a very important and positive stage in someone's life.

When a person's soul mission is complete, they will prepare to discard the physical body – the process of death. During the near-death experience, the return to the physical is always because the soul mission has not yet been accomplished.

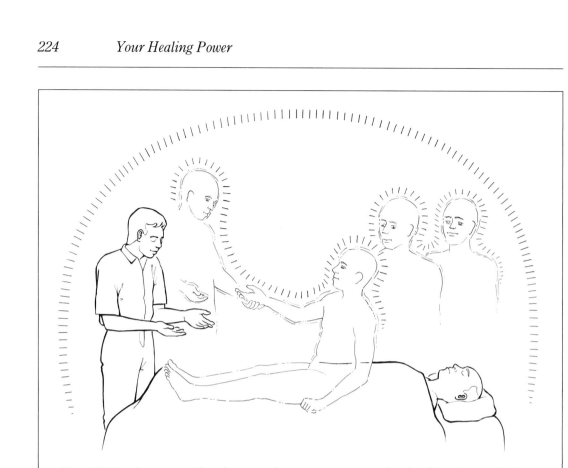

Fig. 53 Passing over. The deceased person sits up in bed in his etheric body. Beings of light come forward to assist him. Spirit healers who have been working with him stand close by.

There are also many reasons why the mission is not carried out before death occurs. The person may not have linked up with their soul mission or the body is breaking down due to damage, abuse or being put in danger. But if the soul no longer wishes to support the body, for whatever reason, it is cast off. When this happens, the link between the subtle bodies and the physical body is broken and the life force ceases to flow into it. The person returns to the etheric level in their etheric body (Fig. 53). All physical pain, disease or disablement is left behind.

PREPARATION FOR DEATH

Most people enter a preparatory stage before death, where they are made aware of their spiritual origins once again. Loved ones on the subtle levels come to visit them and explain to them what will happen when they make the transition from the Earth plane back to the subtle levels. This is why people in terminal conditions are often heard 'talking to themselves' or seem to be seeing others who 'aren't there'. Sometimes these helpers may be encountered in the dream state.

Everything possible is done to help a person get used to the idea of passing over, so that it will not be a shock to the consciousness when it happens. Physical consciousness disappears but all the experiences of that lifetime are recorded in the subconscious mind of the soul. There is actually no death for the soul, but a passing over from one stage of life to another.

From this positive viewpoint it is healthy to contemplate your own death. Death may come when you least expect it. Are you ready? Contemplating your death will help you to see it as part of your life and prepare you for the next stage of your soul journey. First, you need to look at your present life.

EXERCISE 94: Reviewing Your Life

Get a partner to read this exercise or make a tape which you can play back to yourself, allowing pauses where appropriate.

○ Sit in your meditation position. Take three full breaths and relax your body.

○ Review your life, without feelings of regret or remorse, to see what has been accomplished. What are the things you still need to do? Plan how you will achieve this.

○ If there is any unfinished business with anyone, think about how you could clear this up. Is there, for example, any disharmony in your life which you could heal?

○ Have you found a way to help and share with other people?

○ Do you appreciate being you? Do you appreciate those around you? Do you appreciate the planet and all the beings of nature who have been there to share their life with you? Plan how to upgrade your appreciation.

○ Are you in touch with your soul? This is the *you* who will be departing. Each day is precious, your time is precious and your energy is precious. Find ways of acting as if this statement were true for you.

When you have really got in touch with your present life in a positive way, move on to contemplating your own death. Again, the exercise should be read to you or you can put it on tape. Make sure you will not be interrupted.

EXERCISE 95: A Meditation on Death

○ Sit in your meditation position and prepare yourself as in the previous exercise. Put yourself in the hands of your spiritual ideal and ask for protection.

○ For the purpose of the meditation, consider that the time for your death has come. You feel a great sense of peace. Embrace this sense of peace.

○ You are leaving your physical body behind. Now you find yourself travelling towards the light. You can see the light ahead of you.

○ Allow yourself to move into this light and to wait patiently. Let yourself enter into its peace and welcome any experience you will have.

○ When you are ready to come back, thank any being or person whom you have encountered. Come back slowly and gently, back into your physical body. Check that you are aware of your body.

○ Spend time with your experience and make any relevant notes. Do the exercise again whenever you feel the need.

WORKING WITH THE TERMINALLY ILL

Having contemplated your own passing and your life to date, you are in a better position to help others prepare for death. This may mean just being there for them to talk to you about it.

If your work as a healer is with people who are terminally ill, you can be sure that your presence, just quietly giving healing, can bring peace and tranquillity to an atmosphere of fear and anxiety. It is well known that spiritual healing is highly successful in relieving pain. Where drugs are no longer effective or advisable, healers are frequently called in to hospices and terminal wards to help those suffering in this way.

As explained earlier, it is common to hear patients in terminal conditions talking to people whom others cannot see. These are usually loved ones and friends who have already passed over and have come to help them get used to the process of death. If relatives ask you about this, you can reassure them that the patient is not delirious or hallucinating and that it is quite a normal occurrence. I always ask relatives and friends to talk to people who are in a coma as if they *are* present, for on some level they are aware and grateful for this loving response to their unconsciousness.

WORKING WITH HIV AND AIDS PATIENTS

Spiritual healers are having to come to terms with HIV and AIDS. If you have any problems working with people who are HIV positive or who have AIDS, I urge you to speak to those who are working with them, and to study the literature carefully. You may need to realize that you are also being challenged about your fear of death and your attitude to sexuality. In my experience, spiritual healing has a great deal to offer to both groups of people on all levels.

People with AIDS need the spiritual and emotional support which healing can give in a very special way. AIDS is part of someone's soul journey and working with such patients could be part of yours.

COMING TO TERMS WITH BEREAVEMENT

AIDS has brought to our attention the shock and grief which surrounds the death of young people and babies. This is especially felt by parents and friends. You can talk about the healing view of death if *asked* about it. But your main role is to be a channel for healing, so that the dying can use the energy to pass over and the bereaved can use it to cope with the turmoil that they are going through.

Because healing energies have this dual function, healing into death becomes part of most healers' work at some time. This is why it is important for you to address your own feelings about death so that you can work with it from a position of knowledge, confidence and understanding.

For the healer it cannot be a time of sadness or failure because the soul will always use the energies for its own purpose. The death of the physical body is actually a birth into the next stage of life. In this sense it is a time of celebration. It was his new awareness of this process which helped John come to terms with the passing of his mother in Chapter 2.

When somebody dies, they leave a gap in the lives of those who were close to them. The bereaved are often left experiencing a range of feelings, which may include numbness, confusion, anger, loss, sadness, despair and profound grief. Healing can help them to come to terms with their feelings, to accept them and work through them.

When a person has not had this opportunity or has repressed their feelings, they may want to work with the energies they have stored. Again, the healer can help the grieving process through being a good listener, through hands-on healing or working with the chakras, according to what is appropriate.

DEALING WITH UNFINISHED BUSINESS

Some bereaved people are left with unfinished business – something they need to conclude with the deceased. Death leaves them with guilt, anger or pain because they think they have lost the opportunity to do this.

Frank had lost his mother some months before he came to see me. His mother's death had left him numb with shock, but now he was feeling angry because there was so much he still needed to say to her. During the healing, Frank needed help to balance his system and some breathing exercises and a visualization to help him sleep. It took him some time to get in touch with the anger he felt over the unfinished business with his mother, and he said he would like a second session.

Two weeks later, Frank's anger had turned to sadness. Healing was directed to the heart chakra. While he was focused there he became aware of his mother standing as if in front of him. I felt the healing to the heart centre stop and I moved my hand to the solar plexus. Here there was a great deal of activity as Frank burst into tears of bitterness and rage. He clenched his fists and wept. Then, just as suddenly, I needed to move my hand back to the heart chakra. A stream of energy poured into this centre as Frank stopped crying and wiped his eyes. His face became calm and he began to smile faintly. He opened his eyes.

We sat together, quietly, for a few minutes. Later, he was able to tell me how his mother had listened while he told her what a rotten mother she had been and why he felt this. She cried too, he said, and explained how difficult life had been as a mother on her own with three boys to bring up. After allowing each other the space to speak frankly, they were able to be reconciled.

ACHIEVING A NEW RELATIONSHIP

Healers can help the bereaved to temper their loss through a new understanding about the deceased. Loved ones never die in the real sense, neither do they go away. They are simply on another level of experience. A new relationship can begin between the person on the physical and the other on a subtle level.

The bond of love can never be broken unless we want it to be. We can continue in this new way, enriching it with new experience and the awareness that our loved ones are very much all right and very much present. They will find many ways to assure us of their presence and we should not doubt our experiences of this, no matter how strange they may seem to other people.

Such an understanding about the facts of death will bring a new meaning to the concept of the funeral as a way of saying goodbye to the dead and wishing them well in their next phase of life.

DEALING WITH OTHER FORMS OF LOSS

Even if your practice does not bring you into contact with death and the dying, you could still be called upon to deal with the consequences of loss. All change involves loss, and therefore grief, and many other feelings that a person is having to come to terms with. Patients have shown me that people need help with all kinds of loss and that spiritual healing has a role to play here just as it does with the bereaved.

We experience loss not only at the death of a loved one, or a pet, but with events like moving home, changing career, marriage, being made redundant.

Some people are grieving because they feel they have lost their childhood. Very often it is evident that the loss situation presented by a patient embodies a whole pattern of loss which has gone on throughout life.

You will be able to understand how loss is so prominent in human life by looking at your own pattern of loss.

EXERCISE 96: Looking at Your Pattern of Loss

○ Make yourself comfortable and relax the body. Look back over your life and make a careful list of all your losses.

Take your time and note any feelings generated by recalling a particular loss. Have you remembered to include things like losing a treasured item, a friendship, an opportunity, losing touch with someone, going to school for the first time (the 'loss' of mother and home)?

○ Take each loss on your list and consider what strategies you adopted to integrate the loss into your life as you moved forward. If you did not do this, you are still storing the pain of the loss, which will need to be addressed.

Where you have not been able to integrate a loss into your life, you probably felt the pain of its stored energies when you reawakened the memory. The following exercise is one of a number of ways of healing the situation.

EXERCISE 97: Letting Go of Loss

○ First attune yourself as in healing. Locate the pain or disturbed feeling in your body or in the chakra system.

○ Allow yourself to focus on this body part or chakra and wait patiently while the circumstances of the loss are unfolded to your inner vision.

○ When you feel this revelation is complete, breathe love into your heart chakra. Attune from your heart chakra to the situation in your inner vision and see the third side of the Healing Triangle joining with the Source of healing.

○ Put your hands over the body part or chakra where you were focusing and ask for healing for the loss.

○ Wait again as you see the situation healed and are given guidance on what to do.

○ Breathe in and release the energies of the loss situation on the out-breath (if you have not already done so). Keep releasing this way until you feel the loss is cleared for you.

○ Now breathe in healing light to fill the space. Close down in the usual way.

If it seems appropriate, you can extend this exercise to help your patients deal with loss. Remember that this will mean their first accepting the reality of the loss and then feeling the pain of their grief. Care will need to be taken where there is a denial of pain. Give your patient time to address this aspect of loss, even if it means taking another session.

EXERCISE 98: Helping a Partner to Let Go of Loss

○ Attune yourself so that you are ready to heal. Have your partner sit comfortably as if in a healing session.

○ Your partner should take three full breaths and relax the body as you attune to her or him.

○ Ask your partner to identify the loss which s/he wants to deal with, then to focus on the body part or chakra where the pain or discomfort of the loss seems to be located. Your partner should wait patiently while the circumstances of the loss are unfolded to her or him.

○ While s/he is doing this, hold your hands over the part of the body or chakra, being alert and sensitive to the movement of healing energies. You may feel you need to hold your hand over another chakra. If this takes in healing, keep your hand there until the movement of energy ceases.

○ Ask your partner to be guided by inner vision to carry out what needs to be done to bring about the healing. When the movement of energies stops, check with your partner that the inner work has been completed.

○ Now ask your partner to breathe light into the place of focus and release the loss situation on the out-breath. Your partner should close down and visualize the sphere of protection to complete the exercise.

MAINTAINING YOUR OWN ENERGY BALANCE

Working as a healer will involve you in dealing with other people's pain, which may be physical, emotional or mental, and you need to be totally honest with yourself about how you will cope with it. Your response needs to be loving and empathetic, but you should not absorb the pain of others or let their distress become a source of stress in your life. If you carry out the exercises correctly you will avoid this happening. Your clearing, closing down and protection at the end of the day, maintaining your energy balance during the day, are particularly important.

When you start to practise as a healer you may pick up the aches and pains of your patients as you link with them, but this is usually a passing phase and should not persist. If it does, it is an empathetic response which passes once you begin working with your patient.

When you experience this empathetic response outside of the healing room, you should first recall whether you cleared yourself properly after your last patient. (You could be carrying their energies if you forgot to do this.)

If your procedures have been correct, your empathetic response is a signal that you should direct healing to someone who needs it. For example, you may be sitting with a group of people and suddenly feel a pain in your body. Realizing it is not your own, ask for healing to be sent to the person with the condition (sometimes you are shown who it is) and you will notice the pain disappear.

BECOMING A PURE CHANNEL

Some of the exercises in this book will have put you in touch with your own pain about issues you still need to work through or are in the process of working through. Your response to those raised in this chapter, for example, will show you how ready you are to accept the concept of your own soul's journey.

You cannot avoid addressing the effects of your own conditioning and your barriers to personal transformation because any spiritual work you do will bring these to the surface. You will come to recognize that there need to be many little deaths to bring about the internal changes which will allow your true Self to shine through and reveal your healing power.

If your work means development to become a healer, the same process will apply. It is part of the work you need to do on yourself to become as pure a channel as possible for the energies of healing. The conditions which your patients present are the little deaths that they wish to pass through as they journey towards the light.

Your gift to them is to facilitate their letting go of what they no longer need – whether it be ill health, destructive emotions or negative states of mind. Their gift to you is the opportunity to work as a healer.

When you link, with love, to the light that is everywhere – healing must follow.

Useful Addresses

ORGANIZATIONS CONCERNED WITH SPIRITUAL HEALING

British Complementary Medicine
  Association (BCMA)
St Charles Hospital
Exmoor Street
London W10 6DZ

The College of Psychic Studies
16 Queensbury Place
London SW7 2EB

Confederation of Healing
  Organizations (CHO)
The Red and White House
113 High Street
Berkhamsted
Herts HP4 2DJ

The Doctor Healer Network
19 Fore Street
Bishops Steignton
Devon TQ14 9QR

Guild of Spiritual Healers
36 Newmarket
Otley
West Yorks LS21 3AE

Jewish Association of Spiritual
  Healers
10 Wollaton Road
Ferndown
Dorset BH22 8QY

National Federation of Spiritual
  Healers (NFSH)
Old Manor Farm Studio
Church Street
Sunbury-on-Thames
Middx TW16 6RG
*Regional organizations and centres
nationally*

Spiritualist Association of Great
  Britain
33 Belgrave Square
London SW1X 8QL

Spiritualists' National Union
Stansted Hall
Stansted
Essex CM24 8UD

Sufi Healing Order
29 Grosvenor Place
London Road
Bath
Avon BA1 6BA

White Eagle Lodge
New Lands
Brewels Lane
Liss
Hants GU33 7HY

World Federation of Healing
10 The Close
Addington
West Malling
Kent ME19 5BL

TRAINING

Jack and Jan Angelo
Heddfan
1 Lake Villas
Cwmtillery
Gwent NP3 1LU
Wales

College of Healing
Runnings Park
Croft Bank
West Malvern
Worcs WR14 4DU

College of Psychic Studies
16 Queensbury Place
London SW7 2EB

National Federation of Spiritual
  Healers
Old Manor Farm Studio
Church Street
Sunbury-on-Thames
Middx TW16 6RG

Spiritualist Association of Great
  Britain
33 Belgrave Square
London SW1X 8QL

Spiritualists' National Union
Stansted Hall
Stansted
Essex CM24 8UD

White Eagle Lodge
New Lands
Brewells Lane
Liss
Hants GU33 7HY

INTERNATIONAL

For information about organizations
affiliated to the NFSH in Australia,
Canada, Ireland, Israel, New
Zealand, South Africa and the USA
contact the NFSH (see above).

USA

Association for Research and
  Enlightenment (ARE)
PO Box 595
Virginia Beach
VA 23451

Elisabeth Kubler-Ross Center
South Rt 616
Head Waters
VA 24442

JOURNALS CARRYING ARTICLES ON SPIRITUAL HEALING

Caduceus
38 Russell Terrace
Leamington Spa
Warwicks CV31 1HE

Healing Review (Journal of the NFSH)
Old Manor Farm Studio
Church Street
Sunbury-on-Thames
Middx TW16 6RG

Journal of Alternative and Complementary Medicine
Mariner House
53a High Street
Bagshot
Surrey GU19 5AH

Light (Journal of The College of Psychic Studies)
16 Queensbury Place
London SW7 2EB

USA

Venture Inward (Journal of the ARE)
ARE
PO Box 595
Virginia Beach
VA 23451

COUNSELLING

British Association for Counselling
1 Regent Place
Rugby
Warwickshire
CV21 2PJ
Information on counselling and training courses

TO CONTACT THE AUTHOR:

Jack Angelo
Heddfan
1 Lake Villas
Cwmtillery
Gwent NP3 1LU
Wales
UK

Further Reading

Angelo, Jack, *Spiritual Healing: Energy Medicine for Today*, Element Books, Shaftesbury, 1991.

Bach, Edward, *Heal Thyself*, C W Daniel, Saffron Waldon, 1989.

Bendit, L. and Bendit, P., *The Etheric Body of Man*, Theosophical Publishing House, Wheaton, USA, 1977.

Benton, R. G., *Death and Dying*, Van Nostrand, London, 1978.

Bohm, David, *Wholeness and the Implicate Order*, Routledge and Kegan Paul, London, 1981.

Bradshaw, John, *Homecoming: Reclaiming and Championing Your Inner Child*, Piatkus Books, London, 1991.

Brennan, Barbara Ann, *Hands of Light*, Bantam, New York, 1988.

Cade, C. M. and Coxhead, N., *The Awakened Mind: Biofeedback and the Development of Higher States of Awareness*, Dell Publishing, New York, 1979.

Capra, Fritjof, *The Tao of Physics*, Fontana, London, 1983/Berkeley, USA, 1975.
The Turning Point, Fontana, London, 1982/New York, 1982.

Cayce, Edgar, *Auras*, ARE Press, Virginia Beach, USA, 1945.

Cerminara, Gina, *Many Mansions: The Edgar Cayce Story on Reincarnation*, New American Library, New York, 1950/Neville Spearman, London, 1967.

Dhiravamsa, *The Dynamic Way of Meditation*, Turnstone Press, Wellingborough, 1982.

Edwards, Harry, *A Guide to the Understanding and Practice of Spiritual Healing*, The Healer Publishing Company, Guildford, 1974.

Friedman, M. D. and Rosenman, R. H., *Type A Behaviour and Your Heart*, Knopf, New York, 1974.

Gerber, Richard, *Vibrational Medicine*, Bear and Company, Santa Fe, USA, 1988.

Gershom, Rabbi Yonasson, *Beyond the Ashes*, ARE Press, Virginia Beach, USA, 1992.

Grey, Margot, *Return from Death: An Exploration of the Near-Death Experience*, Arkana, London, 1985.

Gurudas, *Flower Essences and Vibrational Healing*, Brotherhood of Life, Albuquerque, USA, 1983.

Hodson, G., *The Miracle of Birth: A Clairvoyant Study of a Human Embryo*, Theosophical Publishing House, Wheaton, USA, 1981.

Kilner, Walter J., *The Human Aura*, Weiser, New York, 1981.

Krystal, Phyllis, *Cutting the Ties that Bind*, Element, Shaftesbury, 1989.

Kubler-Ross, Elisabeth, *On Death and Dying*, Macmillan, London, 1970/ New York, 1969.
Death: The Final Stages of Growth, Prentice Hall, USA, 1978.

Landsdowne, Z., *The Chakras and Esoteric Healing*, Weiser, York Beach, USA, 1986.

Leadbeater, C. W., *The Chakras*, Theosophical Publishing House, Wheaton, USA, 1985.

Levine, Stephen, *Guided Meditations, Explorations and Healings*, Gateway Books, Bath, 1993.

Macbeth, Jessica, *Moon Over Water: The Path of Meditation*, Gateway Books, Bath, 1990.

Maclean, Dorothy, *To Hear the Angels Sing*, Lindisfarne Press, Hudson, USA, 1990.

McGarey, W., *Acupuncture and Body Energies*, Gabriel Press, Phoenix, USA, 1974.

Morse, Melvin, *Closer to the Light*, Bantam Books, London, 1992.
Transformed by the Light, Piatkus Books, London, 1993.

Motoyama, H., *Theories of The Chakras: Bridge to Higher Consciousness*, Theosophical Publishing House, Wheaton, USA, 1981.

Powell, A. E., *The Astral Body*, Theosophical Publishing House, London, 1972.
The Etheric Double, Theosophical Publishing House, London, 1973.

Regush, N. ed., *The Human Aura*, Berkeley Publishing, New York, 1974.

Sechrist, Elsie R., *Death Does Not Part Us*, ARE Press, Virginia Beach, USA, 1992.

Stevenson, Ian, *Children Who Remember Past Lives: A Question of Reincarnation*, University Press of Virginia, USA, 1987.

Tiller, W., *The Kirlian Aura*, Anchor Press, New York, 1974.

Warden, J. William, *Grief Counselling and Grief Therapy*, Routledge, London, 1991.

Watts, Murray and Cooper, Cary L., *Relax: Dealing with Stress*, BBC Books, London, 1992.

White, J., *Kundalini, Evolution and Enlightenment*, Anchor Press, New York, 1979.

Whitton, Joel, *Life Between Life*, Doubleday, New York, 1986.

Glossary

Absent healing – see *distant healing.*

Allopathic – contemporary medicine, particularly medicine using drugs in the treatment of illness.

Astral – the next energy frequency band beyond the etheric. Because emotions are processed in the astral body, it is also known as the *emotional* body.

Aura – the total emanation of the human spirit and various energy bodies which is seen or sensed as a glow of light around the physical body. The human energy field.

Autonomic – the body's automatic regulatory nervous system, divided into the sympathetic and parasympathetic systems.

Avatar – a manifestation of the deity or Source of all energy. Sanskrit, *avatara.*

Bio – prefix referring to anything generated by or part of a living organism.

Chakra – a *subtle* structure, detected in the *etheric* body, designed to allow the flow of *subtle* energies into and out of the human energy field. An energy centre. Sanskrit, *chakram* 'wheel'.

Channel – in healing, a medium for the transmission of healing energies and other high frequency energies. A person who is such a medium. Verb: to act as such a medium or instrument.

Clairvoyant – a person who can perceive or 'see' high frequency energies. Verb: to be clairvoyant is to have well-developed *high sense perception.*

Contact healing – spiritual healing by the laying of hands upon a patient. Hands-on healing.

Distant healing – spiritual healing performed at a distance from the patient. Also known as *absent healing* (in the patient's absence).

Ego – the incarnating personality expressed by the physical consciousness.

Energy – a force directed by and from the Source of all energy.

Energy block – the interruption or cessation of the natural flow of subtle energies through the human system. Often detected as abnormal functioning of one or more chakras.

Etheric – the level of being next to the physical at which energy vibrates at a higher frequency. The preparatory level for entry to and exit from the Earth plane. The first of the subtle bodies.

Guide – in healing, a spirit being from a subtle level, acting as a teacher to an individual or group.

Hands-on healing – see *contact healing*.

Helper – in healing, a spirit being from a subtle level capable of helping a healer in a range of activities, including 'surgical'.

High sense perception – the natural human ability to sense high frequency vibrations as energy patterns which are perceived in the brain as 'seeing', 'hearing', 'feeling', etc – the subtle senses. Sometimes referred to as ESP – extrasensory perception.

Higher Self – the spirit aspect of a human being with direct access to, and contact with, the Source. The embodied aspect of the soul.

Holistic – in therapy, applied to the whole person rather than a specific part or condition. In spiritual healing, the whole person at every level of their being.

Incarnation – birth on the Earth (physical) plane of being. The taking on of a physical body for the spirit to experience this level.

Inner child – general term for an aspect of personality. The wounded child is this aspect damaged by conditioning factors such as parents, childhood trauma, etc. In this book, also an aspect of Self. Inner child work is the therapy of healing, integrating and aligning these two aspects of the human being.

Karma – the law of cause and effect. Imbalances caused in a previous life, or lives, sometimes need to be redressed in this life. Hence, karma should be thought of as a balancing factor, not as retribution.

Kundalini – potential energy of spiritual illumination stored in the base chakra. Activates, unblocks and aligns the chakras. Sanskrit, 'serpent fire'.

Level – a plane of being or experience where matter vibrates at a certain frequency according to the level. A stage of evolution. A state of consciousness.

Life force – the vital energy which is essential to physical life. Sanskrit, *prana*. Chinese, *qi*.

Mental – pertaining to mind. A level of subtle energy beyond the astral which processes thought.

Nadi – a channel for subtle energies.

Out-of-body – the experience of travelling in a subtle body (being out of the physical body), in which a person is not controlled by physical limitations.

Personality – the physical consciousness or self (ego) that tends to see itself as separate from the Source.

Psychic – a subtle sense. Everyone has psychic senses at various stages of development. One who is able to use their psychic senses, such as a healer or medium. Psychic development concerns these senses and should not be confused with *spiritual* development.

Psychic surgery – erroneous term for surgical work carried out at a subtle and/or physical level during certain spiritual healings.

Quantum physics – the branch of physics which studies the energetic characteristics of matter at subatomic levels.

Reincarnation – being born more than once on the Earth plane. The theory (borne out by worldwide research) which proposes this process as a natural part of human life and evolution because all life's lessons cannot be learned in one incarnation. In this book, the theory is not allied to any religious doctrine.

Self – the embodied spirit or soul. Spelt with an initial capital letter to distinguish it from the self (ego). Also Higher Self.

Soul – a specific form of *spirit*, such as a human soul.

Source – in this book, the source of all energy. The Law. The power that is. In religious terms – God, the Creator.

Spirit – the energy of the Source, a soul. A divine spark sent out from the Source on a journey of evolution. All life is spirit. We are spirits (souls) with a body, not bodies with a spirit.

Spiritual – in healing, using energy emanating from the Source specifically to heal. Spiritual activity inclines towards the Source, rather than the limited ego self, to bring about harmony.

Stress – a build up of energy which threatens to overwhelm a system when there is nothing to balance it.

Subtle – of a higher frequency than the physical. Energy travelling at a velocity beyond the speed of light.

Index